THE WONDER DOWN UNDER

THE WONDER DOWN UNDER

THE INSIDER'S GUIDE TO THE ANATOMY, BIOLOGY, AND REALITY OF THE VAGINA

ELLEN STØKKEN DAHL
NINA BROCHMANN, MD

TRANSLATED BY
LUCY MOFFATT

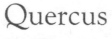

Quercus

New York • London

Quercus

New York • London

ISBN 978-1-68144-021-7
e-ISBN 978-1-68144-019-4

Library of Congress Control Number: 2017960521

Distributed in the United States and Canada by
Hachette Book Group
1290 Avenue of the Americas
New York, NY 10104

This book is not intended as a substitute for the medical advice of physicians. The reader should regularly consult a physician in all matters relating to her health, and particularly in respect of any symptoms that may require diagnosis or medical attention.

Manufactured in the United States

10 9 8 7 6 5 4 3 2 1

www.quercus.com

CONTENTS

Contents

FOREWORD

Unrolling condoms over white polystyrene penises was how we first met. It was early in the fall of 2011 and we were both first-year medical students at the University of Oslo in Norway. We had just signed up to become volunteer sex education teachers with an organization run by medical students. With slippery fingers smelling of synthetic lube, we had no idea that this encounter, and the budding friendship that came out of it, would culminate in a project that would ultimately expand far outside of little Oslo, reaching readers across the world. We were just two curious and enthusiastic nerds, eager to impart knowledge about proper condom technique.

The next couple of years, we traveled around Norway as sex-ed teachers, working with groups of teenagers, sex workers, and refugees. We were teaching them the essentials about their bodies and a healthy sex life. We drew ovaries and testicles on chalkboards, discussed sexual consent through role-playing exercises, and had teenagers create their personal wish list for their sexual debut. It was a wonderful and meaningful job, but we were overwhelmed by the amount of questions and concerns people had. There is so much anxiety, shame, and insecurity connected to our most intimate body parts. Sometimes it feels like we could have spent a whole day just answering questions. *Do I look normal down there? Does discharge mean I have a sexually transmitted disease? How can I ensure that I'll bleed on my wedding night?* After a while, it just didn't feel like we were doing enough. If we were to answer each of these questions in person, it would take a lifetime.

Our solution was to start a blog called *Underlivet* (*The Genitals*), to reach a larger audience. We wanted to give girls and women a sense of wonder and pride in their incredible bodies. Our goal was to provide sound, research-based medical information, written in an accessible and funny way. No moralism, no embarrassment, just honest and trustworthy information.

In a very short time, *Underlivet* became one of the most read health blogs in Norway, and we mustered the courage to write the book you are holding in your hands right now. *The Wonder Down Under* came out in Norwegian in January 2017 and now, less than a year later, it is being translated into thirty languages, from Korean to Polish, from Russian to Dutch. It is fantastic—and slightly terrifying—to be able to spread one's debut book to so many people. We are happy to know that women and girls in all corners of the world will get to read what we have to say, because we strongly believe that good sexual health is critical. At the same time, the overwhelming interest in our book also saddens us, because it shows us that information on female sexual health is scarce. It demonstrates that women all over the world have serious questions and few resources to turn to. We wish the reality were different, but it shouldn't have come as a surprise. Scandinavia is, after all, known for its openness regarding sexuality, so if *we* have these questions, everybody else must have them too.

The American edition of *The Wonder Down Under* has been adapted and revised to provide relevant information to North American readers. Men and boys will certainly find invaluable (and most likely surprising) information contained here, but it's you women we're writing this book for—especially all the ladies out there who are unsure whether your bodies are working the way they should, whether you look the way you should, and whether you feel the way you should. We hope this book will give you the confidence you need. We're also writing for all of you who are happy and proud but want to learn more about the amazing organ between your legs. This intimate body part of ours is incredible, and we believe much of the key to good health (sexual and otherwise) lies in understanding how the body works—in understanding the wonder down under.

* * *

When women make choices about their own bodies and sexuality, they do so within a larger context. Cultural, religious, and political forces regulate these choices, whether it's a matter of contraception, abortion, sexual identity, or sexual practices. In autumn 2016, for instance, we read newspaper articles about the hypersexualized behavior of teenagers in some Norwegian high schools.[1] Merciless social pressure to fit in meant that sixteen-year-old girls were feeling compelled to overstep their own sexual boundaries—so drastically in some cases that we could scarcely believe what we were reading. It's hair-raising that some eighteen-year-old boys think it's okay to use their social status as upperclassmen to get freshmen girls to give blow jobs to ten boys in a row, but that is exactly what was happening. As Norwegian newspaper *VG* wrote at the time, this is a culture in which "the distinction between consensual sex and assault has grown dangerously thin."[2] In recent decades, we have seen the increasing sexualization of youth culture, particularly of girls—and not just in Norway, but all over the world. For many young women, unfortunately, growing up in this environment involves enduring a string of unpleasant sexual experiences that they then struggle with later in life. It shouldn't be this way.

We want women to be able to make independent choices, with all the facts on the table; we want their choices to be based on medical knowledge, not gossip, misunderstandings, and fear. A good knowledge base about how the body works will make it easier for women to make their own choices with self-confidence and self-assurance. Sexuality and sexual health must be demystified, and we must take ownership of our bodies. The intention of this book is to give you the opportunity to make sensible and well-informed choices that suit *you*.

Perhaps you're wondering: Why should I bother reading a medical book written by two Norwegian students? One of them hasn't even finished medical school yet! Even as we were writing the manuscript for the Norwegian edition of this book, we asked ourselves that very same question plenty of times. We are neither fully trained doctors nor experts in any way whatsoever. We therefore approached the creation of this book, and particularly foreign editions of it, with a healthy dose of humility.

We took courage from the example of German medical student Giulia Enders. She achieved resounding success with her book *Darm mit Charme* (published in English as *Gut: The Inside Story of Our Body's Most Underrated Organ*), which transformed intestines and feces into topics people could discuss on prime-time talk shows. The rhyming title of our book is an homage to the German title of her book. She paved the way for us, showing how medicine can be made understandable and funny, and—more important—how we can talk about our most intimate body parts without even a whiff of shame.

As medical students, we have one advantage that nobody can take away from us: We are curious, we are young, and we have the nerve to ask the "stupid" questions—often because we're wondering about the same things ourselves, or because our friends are. We don't have professional reputations to jeopardize and we haven't (yet) spent so much time among the ranks of doctors that we've forgotten how to speak plainly to people. We hope more of our young colleagues will act on the urge to write.

Many times, when we were working on the book, we found there were things we'd totally misunderstood. We, too, had fallen victim to the myths surrounding the female sex organs. And there are a lot of these myths. The ones about the hymen are perhaps the most persistent, and continue to place girls at risk the whole world over. Yet few doctors trouble themselves about this little body part. Certain doctors even help perpetuate the myths by checking girls' genitals on behalf of their parents. In our quest for answers, we often found that senior gynecologists would brush aside our questions about the hymen as uninteresting or unimportant. This is incomprehensible, given the implications the hymen can have in many women's lives. Our TEDxOslo talk, "The Virginity Fraud," which debunks the most common misconceptions about the hymen, has been seen over two million times at the date of publication, and our inboxes continue to be filled with personal stories from women who have experienced the consequences of these anatomical fallacies.

Another myth is that hormonal contraception is unnatural and dangerous. This misconception leads to unplanned pregnancies for thousands of girls and women who choose to use unsafe contraceptive methods instead. We understand that people are confused and afraid of the side effects, and we are sick and tired of seeing people in the medical community dismiss concerns without providing proper explanations. That is why we decided to set aside plenty of space in the book for a thorough discussion of contraception. We review the most important research on possible side effects, such as mood swings and low libido. Where there is uncertainty, we are open about it, but our primary aim is to reassure you. Serious side effects are in fact extremely rare, and there is little to indicate that depression or a decreased sex drive are problems that affect a large proportion of women using hormonal contraceptives. There are always exceptions, but we hope that after reading this book you'll be able to distinguish between what is usual and what is unusual.

Other myths are not directly harmful, but reflect the fact that even when it comes to medical research this has been a man's world for far too long. When friends complain that they never have "vaginal orgasms," this shows how much our understanding of female sexuality has been colored by men's needs over the centuries. There is no "vaginal orgasm" as such, just orgasms as a result of different types of stimulation, all of which are equally delightful. We hope that women can stop feeling inferior for needing other forms of stimulation beyond penetration in order to achieve orgasm.

These are just a few of the many things you will read about in *The Wonder Down Under*. We hope you're looking forward to joining us on a journey through the female sex organs, from the vulva to the ovaries. Hopefully you'll learn lots, just as we did while working on the book. The most important thing for us is that after reading this book you'll be able to relax. A body is just a body. We all have one, and it will offer us joys and challenges alike throughout our life. Be proud of what your body achieves and be patient with it when it struggles.

Ellen Støkken Dahl
Nina Brochmann, MD
Oslo, Norway

PART 1: THE GENITALS

Our genital area is, perhaps, our most intimate body part. It is our close companion from the moment we burst into the world from our mother's womb and first see the light of day. In nursery school we delighted in comparing innie and outie "pee-pees" as we were first becoming aware of our bodies. Then, with the onset of puberty, came the first dark hairs on our pubic areas. We all remember our first period, whether the moment was filled with pride or terror. Perhaps you began to masturbate and found you could make your body curl up in pleasure. Then came your sexual debut, with all that entails in the way of vulnerability, curiosity, and desire. Perhaps you have had children and have experienced the enormous changes your sex organs undergo, and the miracles they are capable of performing. No matter your experience to this point, one thing is certain: your genitals are part of you. It's time you got to know them better.

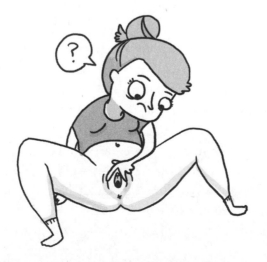

VULVA—THE WONDER DOWN UNDER

Stand naked in front of the mirror and take a good look at yourself. Your genital area begins low down on your belly, with a fatty area that covers the very front of your hipbone. This soft area is called the Venus mound, and it becomes covered in hair during puberty. The fatty cushion on the Venus mound is larger for some women than others, so some people's pubic areas protrude slightly from their belly, whereas others have flatter variants. Both are perfectly normal.

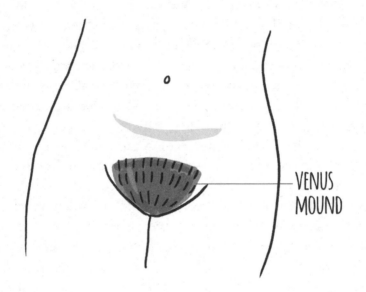

If you run your gaze down your Venus mound, you come to what we call the vulva, though it may also be called the pussy, hoo-ha, snatch, vag, cunt, and any number of other euphemisms. We Norwegians also call it the mouse. *Vulva* may not be the world's most commonly used word, but if you're a woman and take a look between your legs, what you'll find there is your vulva.

A lot of people think the visible part of the female sex organs is the vagina. "There's hair growing on my vagina," you might say, or "You have such a lovely vagina," but actually that's not right. The vagina doesn't have any hair and it isn't especially easy to see it, although it is of course totally lovely. *Vagina* is just the name for a part of your sexual apparatus, more accurately the muscular tube you use when you have penetrative sex or give birth—in other words, the tube that leads up to the uterus. The reason we're focusing on terminology is that our sex organs are about so much more than just the vagina, no matter how much pleasure we get out of it! Most people who refer to the female genitalia as the vagina actually mean the vulva, and it's the vulva we'll begin with in our description of the fantastic female sex organs.

The vulva is formed like a flower, with two layers of petals. And believe it or not, it wasn't us who came up with the flower metaphor. When looking at the different parts of the vulva, it makes sense to start from the outside and work our way in.

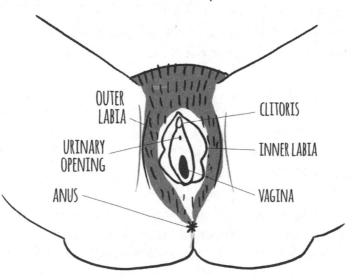

The purpose of the petals, or *labia* (the Latin word for *lips*), is to protect the sensitive parts that lie farther in. The outer labia, which are thicker than the inner ones, are full of fat and work a little like air bags or shock absorbers. Although they may be long enough to cover the inner labia, they can also be very short. Some people just have two small dents in their skin that frame the rest of the vulva on either side.

The outer labia are covered in regular skin. Like the rest of the skin on your body, it's full of sebaceous glands, sweat glands, and hair follicles. In addition to hair, which is a great thing, it is also possible to get pimples and eczema on your outer labia, which isn't so great. Sadly, skin will be skin.

The inner labia are often longer than the outer labia, although not necessarily. They may be full of crinkles and folds, like a skirt made of tulle. When you stand looking at yourself in the mirror, it's possible your inner labia may protrude markedly from your outer labia. Other people may have to spread aside their outer labia in order to see their inner labia.

In contrast to the fatty outer labia, the inner labia are thinner and highly sensitive. They aren't as sensitive as the clitoris, which is the most sensitive place on your body, but they are full of nerve endings, so it can feel very good to touch them.

The inner labia don't have regular skin. Instead, they are covered with a mucous membrane—you've seen mucous membranes before, for example on the outer surface of your eyeball and inside your mouth. These organs are simply covered with a protective and moistening layer of mucus. Regular skin is covered in a layer of dead skin cells, sort of like a duvet cover consisting of dead relatives. This dead layer provides protection, and regular skin thrives in dry conditions. However, mucous membranes do not have a protective layer of dead skin cells, and are therefore less resistant to wear and tear. For example, long inner labia may become sore if they chafe against tight jeans. Unlike regular skin, mucous membranes prefer to be moist. There is no hair on mucous membranes, which means that there isn't any hair on the part of the vulva inside your outer labia either.

If you spread aside your inner labia, you'll find the area known as the vestibulum. *Vestibulum* comes from Latin and means "vestibule," which is the area between the entrance to a building and its interior. If you're not the kind of person who goes to the theater or the opera, the vestibule is the place where you drink champagne during the intermission. It's the splendid entrance hall with columns and soft red velvet curtains. The female vestibulum doesn't have any columns to speak of, but it's an entranceway nonetheless, and we would argue that it has the same velvety grandeur. You'll find two holes here: the urinary and the vaginal openings. The urinary opening lies between the clitoris, which is located right at the front, where the labia meet, and the vagina, which is closer to the anus.

Few people have a conscious relationship to their urinary opening, even though we all use it multiple times a day. In fact, some people don't realize there is a separate hole for urine, and think that we're like men, who have just one hole for two things: in a man's case, sperm and urine. Be assured, that isn't the case: the urethra has its own opening. We don't pee with our vaginas, although it's easy to misunderstand this, even if you've seen your share of female genitalia. The urinary opening can be very difficult to find even if you look for it with a mirror. The urethra is quite tiny and there are often a lot of small folds of skin around the hole, but she who seeks shall eventually find.

VAGINA—THE AMAZING EXPANDING TUBE

Unlike the little urinary opening, the much larger vaginal opening should be easy to find. The vagina is a narrow, muscular tube seven to ten centimeters in length, which leads from the vulva to the uterus. Most of the time this tube is compressed so that the back and front walls are squeezed up against each other. This helps keep you waterproof. Imagine that!

When you get turned on, your vagina expands both lengthwise and breadthwise; it's also highly elastic in all directions. It's a bit like a pleated skirt. If you examine it with your fingers, you'll notice how ridged it feels.

The muscles around the vagina are strong, which you'll see if you stick a finger into your vagina and then clench it tight. Like other muscles, these—the pelvic floor muscles—get stronger when you exercise them.

The inside of the vagina is covered with a moist mucous membrane. Most of the moisture seeps straight through the vaginal walls from the interior of the body, rather than being produced in glands. There are no glands in the vaginal wall itself, although a small amount of secretion comes from glands in the cervix. There is always moisture present in the vagina, but when you get turned on, you become even wetter than usual because more fluid soaks in through the vaginal wall when extra blood flows to the whole of the genital area. You'll notice the increased blood supply to your genitals because your erectile tissue (yes, you have erectile tissue, more about that later) will become engorged. The fluid produced when you're aroused reduces the friction in your vagina when you masturbate or have penetrative sex. Less friction means less damage to the mucus membrane on the vulva and on the vaginal wall, which can often take quite a pummeling during sex. It's not unusual to feel a bit sore or to experience some bleeding from small tears in the vaginal wall after sex, but, luckily, it's quite harmless. The vaginal wall is good at repairing itself.

In addition to the moisture that comes through the vaginal wall, some mucus also comes from two glands located in the vestibulum. They're behind the vaginal opening, toward your butt, with one on either side. They are called Bartholin's glands after the seventeenth-century Danish anatomist, Caspar Bartholin the Younger. They produce a slick fluid that helps lubricate the vaginal opening. Bartholin's glands are oval-shaped, the size of peas, and can be troublemakers. If the little tube through which they dispatch their mucus gets blocked, it can result in a vulval cyst. This is detectable as a small, hard lump on one side of the vulva, like a little balloon. If this sort of cyst becomes infected, it can turn into a painful business, but the problem can be fixed with minor surgery. There is some disagreement over how important Bartholin's glands are for lubrication of the vagina.[1] Women who have the glands removed as a result of problems with cysts and infections still experience an increase in vaginal moisture when they're turned on.

On the anterior vaginal wall, in other words toward the bladder, lies a spot that is popular in the sex columns of women's magazines.

We're talking about the G-spot. The area got its name from the German gynecologist Ernst Gräfenberg, who discovered it. Although researchers have been discussing and searching for the G-spot since the 1940s, it's still pretty controversial—researchers are uncertain what it is, and its existence as a separate entity hasn't even been proven.

The G-spot is described as an extra-sensitive point in some women's vaginas, and certain women say they can achieve orgasm just by stimulating it. The G-spot apparently lies a bit into the vagina on the anterior vaginal wall, toward the stomach, and can be stimulated by making a "come hither" gesture with a finger. Imagine a Disney witch trying to lure you toward her—that's the movement you're after. According to some women's descriptions, stimulation of the G-spot feels better than or different from stimulation elsewhere in the vagina. As you may have noticed, the vagina itself is not particularly sensitive compared with the vulva and especially the clitoris. Sensitivity is highest in the vaginal opening and lessens farther up.

The media often treats the G-spot as if it were a separate anatomical structure. It is especially easy to gain this impression if you read sex columns or sexual self-help books. A British article from 2012 reviewed the existing research on the G-spot as a separate area of the vagina and concluded that the proof was sparse. Most G-spot research is based on questionnaires in which women describe it themselves. The article also showed that many of the women who believe in the G-spot have difficulty pointing it out on themselves. The researchers also reported that studies based on imaging techniques have failed to find any separate structure capable of producing orgasm or sexual pleasure in women, other than the clitoris.[2]

One hypothesis about the G-spot is that, in fact, it is not a separate physical structure but simply a deep-lying inner part of the clitoris that is stimulated during sex, directly through the vaginal wall. In 2010, a group of researchers published a study in which they had observed the anterior vaginal wall of a woman while she had vaginal sex with her partner. They used ultrasound to see what was happening and search for the G-spot. They didn't find it, but concluded that the inner parts of the clitoris lie so close to the anterior vaginal wall that the clitoris may be the answer to the G-spot mystery.[3]

Some studies claim that the G-spot is important for achieving a squirting orgasm,[4] and this leads us to another theory. The G-spot may be linked to a group of glands that are located between the urethra and the anterior vaginal wall. Known as Skene's glands, they are the female equivalent of the male prostate, a walnut-size gland that surrounds the urethra between the bladder and the penis. Skene's glands are associated with female ejaculation, or squirting orgasms, as they produce liquid that may be released during orgasm—just like the prostate.

It's odd that an area as accessible as the vaginal wall should be so shrouded in mystery—especially when there's so much speculation about the G-spot. We wait with bated breath for more high-quality research on the female body.

CLITORIS—AN ICEBERG

Perhaps you were surprised just now to read about the "inner parts" of the clitoris. What inner parts? After all, as we usually describe it, the clitoris is the size of a raisin and is located on the uppermost part of the vulva, neatly positioned at the point where the inner labia meet. But this little button is actually just the tip of an iceberg. In the deep darkness of the pelvic area, an organ lies hidden that exceeds all your wildest imaginings.

Although anatomists have known since the 1800s that the clitoris is a largely subterranean organ,* this is far from general knowledge. While the male penis is described in detail in anatomies and textbooks, the clitoris has remained a curiosity. As late as 1948, the influential medical textbook *Gray's Anatomy* chose not to label

---

* The German anatomist Georg Ludwig Kobelt described the inner construction of the clitoris in the 1840s and concluded that male and female sexual organs shared the same building blocks.

the clitoris. Nor has the male-dominated medical world been particularly interested in conducting further research on that particular organ. There is still disagreement over what actually forms the parts of the clitoris and how it works. In a medical context, this is startling.

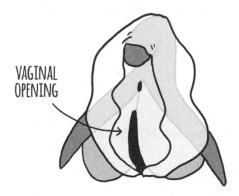

VAGINAL
OPENING

What we do know is that what most people describe as the clitoris is only a fraction of a large organ that extends into the pelvis and down along either side of the vulva.[5, 6, 7] If we had X-ray glasses, we would see that the clitoris complex is shaped like an upside-down Y. The little raisin, called the glans or "head" of the clitoris, is right at the top. It may be from 0.5 to 3.5 centimeters long, but it appears smaller because it is partly covered by a little hood.[8] The head of the clitoris is its only visible part. Below that is a shaft, which descends through the body at an angle, like a boomerang, before the shaft splits into two legs, which lie on either side of the genital area, buried beneath the labia.

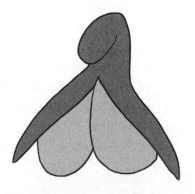

Each of the legs contains erectile tissue, the corpus cavernosum, which fills with blood and becomes engorged during arousal. Between these two legs there are two extra bodies of erectile tissue, the bulbi vestibuli or *vestibular bulbs*, which surround the vaginal and urinary openings.

For those of you who were especially attentive in your high school health class, this description may be ringing some bells—but wasn't it the man's penis that had a head, shaft, and erectile tissue? The principal source of female pleasure, the clitoris, is a well-kept secret, in stark contrast to the erect penis, which is conspicuous, to say the least. It may therefore seem surprising that the clitoris and the penis are two versions of the same organ.

Up until about the twelfth week in the uterus, the genital tracts of male and female embryos are exactly alike, dominated by a kind of mini-penis (or giga-clitoris!) known as the genital tubercle. It has the potential to develop into either a female or male sexual organ. Since the penis and the clitoris both develop from the same basic structure, the two organs share many similarities of form and function.

The head of the penis is actually the same as the clitoral button, and that is why both are given the same name, *glans*. The glans is the most sensitive spot on both the female and male body. It is estimated that the female and male glans both contain more than 8,000 sensory nerve endings. A sensory nerve ending receives information about pressure and touch, and sends signals onward to the brain, where the information is interpreted as either pain or pleasure. The more nerve endings there are, the more nuanced and powerful the signals the brain receives. Nonetheless, the head of the clitoris is a great deal more sensitive than the head of the penis because the nerve endings are concentrated into a much smaller area—in fact, the concentration is fifty times higher![9]

Unfortunately, the perception of the clitoris as a pleasure button may have led some men to believe that all pressure is good pressure. If a bit of light pressure doesn't elicit the desired result, they simply press harder and harder. But that's not how the clitoris works. Since it is so rich in nerve endings, even the tiniest variation in touch is perceptible. Although this offers undreamt-of possibilities for stimulation and pleasure, it also means that the transition to pain or outright numbness can be rapid. Over the long term, hard pressure can cause the nerve endings to simply refuse to send signals to the brain: the clitoral button is switched to "mute." If that happens, the clitoris has to be left in peace until it's ready to start talking again. In other words, it's a bit like dating: if you try too hard, things often go wrong.

A man's erectile tissues make the penis hard when they become engorged with blood. Women's erectile tissues do exactly the same thing to the clitoris. When we are aroused, the clitoral complex can swell to double its normal size.[10] It is, quite simply, an impressive erection. Since the clitoral legs and the bulbi vestibuli lie beneath the labia and around the urinary and vaginal openings, this can make the vulva look larger during arousal. In addition, the vestibulum and the inner labia take on a darker, purplish-red coloring thanks to the blood that gathers there.

The similarities between the penis and the clitoris don't stop there. Men like to boast about "morning wood" and nightly erections, but women get them, too. In a study conducted at the University of Florida in the 1970s, two women with large clitorises were studied and compared with men. The study found that the women had just as many nightly "erections" during deep sleep as the men did.[11] Another study found that women had "erections" up to eight times a night, for a combined period of one hour and twenty minutes on average![12]

As you'll have gathered by now, there's a lot you didn't learn about the clitoris in your high school health class. This proud organ has been overlooked, undervalued, and hidden away for far too long. Only when we realize how the clitoris extends to encompass all areas of our pelvic region can we understand what a marvelous instrument of pleasure we're equipped with.

BLOODY VIRGINITY

For thousands of years, different cultures have been extremely concerned with virginity—and usually just women's, not men's. A man cannot be a Madonna or a whore, pure or impure, but a woman can, and "luckily" vaginal bleeding on the wedding night can reveal what kind of a woman she is.

A lot of people use the term "pop her cherry" as if a woman who hasn't had sex before can be popped like a bottle of champagne; as if her vagina is as different before and after her sexual debut as a bottle of Moët & Chandon is with and without its cork. As you may have gathered from our tone here, that is not the case.

The topic of virginity is widespread in popular culture. For the vampire Jessica in the HBO show *True Blood*, who was a virgin when she was turned, every sex act is like her first, and she has to bleed time after time. Doubt surrounds the queen Margaery Tyrell in *Game of Thrones*. Is she really still *pure* after marrying king number three? The CW show *Jane the Virgin* focuses heavily on the lead character's decision to stay a virgin until marriage, even after having a child via accidental IVF.

Even our classics in Norway describe virginity and bleeding. "Damn!" Kristin Lavransdatter, heroine of a Nobel prize–winning historical fiction trilogy, could have said as the blood ran down her thighs in the film we saw in our Norwegian classes. Instead, she said something along the lines of, "Who will want a flower whose bloom has been ripped off?" She wept bitterly in the arms of her lover, Erlend, who had no need to weep himself. As a man, he had no virtue to lose. The idea that a woman is an innocent flower, and that "taking" her virginity is the same as ripping the head off a flower is even encoded in medical language. The bleeding that is supposed to occur when a woman has sex for the first time is called "deflowering."[13]

The systems and traditions for controlling women's bodies are ancient and widespread, and language plays an important supporting role in encoding them in culture. Of course, there's no equivalent euphemism for men losing their virginity.

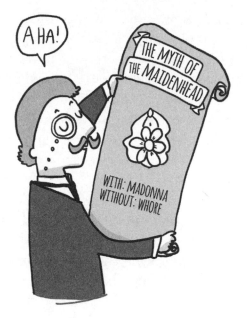

As you may have gathered, it's time to talk about the hymen, that mythical structure in the vaginal opening that still costs women the world over their honor—or even their lives—based solely on antiquated traditions and misinformation. It's unbelievable that men and women are still differentiated in this way—that something as wonderful and positive as sex should mean ruin for a woman without having any consequences for a man.

The hymen has traditionally been presented as a kind of seal of chastity that, as myth has it, will be broken and bleed when a woman first has sexual intercourse (and only then). This bleeding has been used as proof of virginity—a proof so important for people that it used to be customary to hang the bloodstained sheet out to dry after the wedding night, so that the whole neighborhood could see that everything had been as it should.

The myth of the hymen says: If you bleed after sexual intercourse, people will know that you haven't had sex before. If you don't bleed, you've already had sex. But this myth, like most others, is totally wrong.

The belief is perpetuated by the widespread perception of the hymen as a membrane. When you hear the word *membrane* perhaps you picture a taut sheet of plastic wrap that will split if you poke a hole in it. *Pop!* But if you've ever looked at your genitalia in a mirror, you'll know there isn't a sheet of plastic in your vagina, even if you haven't had sex before. Lately we've heard a lot of talk to the effect that "the hymen doesn't exist." But let's not allow one myth to be replaced by another. While it's true there isn't a seal keeping the vagina shut, that doesn't mean there isn't an anatomical structure that is the cause of the misunderstanding. The hymen exists, all right.

Just inside the vaginal opening is an encircling fold of mucous membrane, which lies up against the vaginal wall like a ring. This little ring is what has traditionally been called the virginal membrane, the maidenhead, and such. We also call it the hymen. Although these words all mean the same thing, *virginal membrane* is such a misleading term that it is better to avoid it.

All women are born with a hymen, but that doesn't mean it's any use to you. The hymen is the female equivalent of male nipples. It has no function and is just a leftover from our embryonic existence.

The hymen has both depth and breadth. In other words, it isn't thin like plastic wrap, but thick and robust. In prepubescent girls, it is usually smooth and shaped like a doughnut with a hole in the middle. Then the body's hormonal orchestra takes the stage and, like so many other parts of the body, the hymen changes during puberty. By the time puberty ends, it has often become crescent shaped. It is broadest at the rear, toward the anus, and still encircles the vaginal wall, but now it has a bigger hole in the center.[14] That's how it is in theory at least. In reality, there's no single way a hymen should look.

Most women have a circular hymen with a hole in the middle, but not everybody's is even and smooth. The hymen is often wrinkled and indented; this is not a sign of sexual activity. Some people have hymens with strands stretched across the vaginal opening, so that they look more like an ø (a vowel we use in Norwegian) than an *o*. Others have hymens that look like sieves, with lots of small holes instead of one big hole in the middle, or hymens that just look like small fringes on the vaginal wall. A small minority of girls have a hymen that does actually cover the whole entrance to the vagina. These girls often have a fairly rigid, tough hymen, and this is a variant that spells trouble, because of course menstrual blood has to have a way out! Women with this type of hymen will often only discover the problem when they have their first period. If the menstrual blood gets trapped inside the vagina, it can cause severe pain and require surgery. This rare variant is the closest we get to the myth of the hymen as a seal.[15]

Whatever form the hymen takes, it is flexible and elastic, except in those very few cases where it covers the entire opening. Even so, the hymen is the narrowest point of the vagina. The vagina has a dramatic ability to expand and then contract again; you can, after all, get a baby through it. But although the hymen is elastic, it's not necessarily elastic enough for sexual intercourse. It's a bit like a rubber band that can be stretched to a certain length but snaps if you pull too hard on it.

When you have vaginal sex for the first time, the hymen is stretched along with the rest of the vagina. For many women the hymen is elastic enough to not sustain any injury, but for others, the hymen can tear and bleed a little. In other words, some women bleed the first time they have sex and others don't. It all depends on the shape and elasticity of their hymen. Women who have an unusual-shaped hymen with a part that stretches across the vaginal opening will find that this part may tear to make way for a penis or fingers.

It's difficult to be certain just how many women have hymens that bleed when they have sex for the first time. There's some statistical material, but the numbers vary. Two different studies we've looked at reported that 56 percent or 40 percent of all women, respectively, bleed when they have consensual vaginal sex for the first time. Those numbers are far from all women, but still a high proportion.[16, 17]

These studies involved interviewing women about the first time they had sexual intercourse, so we can't possibly know for sure whether it was the hymen that bled, even though the hymen is the vagina's narrowest point, or whether the blood came from elsewhere. As we noted earlier in the section about the vagina, it's both possible and normal for bleeding to occur as a result of small tears in the vaginal wall if people have even slightly rough sex, aren't wet enough, or tense up the muscles in their vagina because they're nervous. This can happen the first time people have sex or on several occasions.

Another important part of the myth about the hymen involves virginity tests. These tests mean people believe it is possible to tell from looking at a woman's genitalia whether or not she has had sexual intercourse. Joan of Arc underwent a virginity test, and so have a whole load of women from different conservative environments in modern times.

Now and then, we hear about doctors who are still carrying out virginity tests on young women at the incitement of their parents, who want proof that their daughters are intact[18]—despite the fact that experts in forensic medicine deem such tests to be irrelevant.[19] We also hear of doctors issuing virginity certificates to terrified young women who are afraid of the consequences if there's no bleeding on the wedding night. None of this is common practice in the United States, and virginity testing is largely considered irrelevant to medical health.[20]

It turns out that it is usually impossible to see any difference between the hymens of girls who have had sex and those who haven't.[21,22] In fact, the World Health Organization has said that "there is no place for virginity (or 'two-finger') testing; it has no scientific validity." And although the hymen may be damaged during sexual intercourse if it's severely stretched, the damage won't necessarily be permanent. It turns out that in many cases the hymen can heal without any visible scarring.[23]

Much of the research on the hymen and the way it changes after a woman's sexual debut comes from surveys of women and girls who have been exposed to sexual abuse. A Norwegian review article reports that what were previously thought to be suspect changes in children's hymens—for example a wide opening[24] or narrow brim—are now interpreted as entirely non-specific findings and not as proof of sexual abuse.[25] These variations in the hymen can also be found among children who haven't been exposed to sexual abuse. The authors of the article are, incidentally, careful to note that the lack of a relevant finding doesn't prove that a child has *not* been exposed to sexual abuse.

On the whole, you can't find out whether or not a woman has had sex by looking between her legs. The hymen is not the preserve of those who haven't had sex, nor is there one variant of hymen for those who've had sex and another for those who are still "virgins." Like other body parts, the hymen's appearance varies according to the individual. Sorry, but virginity tests don't work.

Unfortunately, this knowledge about the hymen is not generally known. In rare cases, women still resort to surgery to guarantee that they'll bleed on their wedding night—hymenoplasty, as it's called. In Norway, a private clinic in Oslo offered this surgery until as recently as 2006.[26] It stopped carrying out hymenoplasties after seeking the Council for Medical Ethics' view on the practice. The council objected to the procedure because it becomes a kind of quick fix or replacement for a proper solution to the problem: cultural change.[27]

Hymenoplasty still exists as a strictly elective plastic surgery procedure—even in the United States, where no statistics on frequency are kept. On the Internet, you can buy fake membranes containing theatrical blood for thirty dollars, which guarantee that you can "kiss your deep dark secret goodbye" and get married with confidence.[28] Incidentally, Egyptian politicians suggested prohibiting imports of the product in 2009.[29]

Why do we choose to resort to these kinds of solutions instead of informing people that the absence of bleeding does not equate to the absence of virginity? And why is it so important for some of us to have proof that women remain "intact" until they get married? The bleeding must become less significant and virginity tests must be abandoned once and for all, but most important, we must jettison the idea that virginity itself is important.

The problem is that it is difficult to find reliable information about the hymen—and, not least, to distinguish what is right from what is less right or just plain wrong. In our quest for knowledge about the hymen, we found little information that was accessible, available to most people, and also correct. We found a great deal of research literature, but the hymen is barely mentioned in the gynecological textbooks that are most commonly used in medical school, and even there some of the myths are repeated. We still have tons of questions. Doctors have shown disappointingly little interest in a structure that can, in the worst of cases, cause modern women to lose their honor or their lives. Worse still, the little information that is actually available doesn't reach the people who need it most.

THE OTHER HOLE

"Where the sun don't shine," we say, when we talk about the butthole. This crinkly, brown orifice is often overlooked in discussions about women's genitals, but the vagina and the rectum are only separated by a thin wall. Being in such close quarters, the butthole is unavoidably connected to the vagina, the vulva, and many women's sexual self-image.

The butthole, also called the *anus*, is a formidable ring of muscle designed to keep feces in place until we're ready to get rid of them. This has clearly been a vital task from time immemorial, as our body comes equipped with not just one but two sphincters in a row. If one of them lets us down, we have an extra backup.

The inner sphincter is controlled by what we call the autonomous nervous system, which is the part of the nervous system we don't have conscious control over. When the body notices that the rectum is beginning to fill up with feces, signals go out telling the inner sphincter to relax. This is the defecation reflex, which we experience as a sudden urge to find the nearest toilet.

If we had only this primitive reflex, we would be pooping all the time, the way infants and toddlers do, but we humans are social creatures, and we learn to control when and where we defecate as we get older. The outer sphincter—the one you can feel if you put a finger in your butt and clench—is the top dog. It's a voluntary muscle, which ensures that you can hold off until circumstances allow you a little privacy. If you keep clenching for long enough, your body takes the hint and the primal instincts realize they've lost. The feces discreetly withdraw back up into the colon and patiently await a better occasion. The poo window, as we like to call it, has closed for the time being.

The butt is the dark corner of the genital area, but fortunately there's more to it than just crap. The area around and just inside the anus is full of nerve endings just waiting to be stimulated. Some people find it expands the dimensions of their sex life if they invite their butt to join the party. Others may content themselves with acknowledging that the butt is a beautiful system, and sending it a few affectionate thoughts from time to time.

HAIRY TIPS

Being human means having hair on your crotch (as far as nature's concerned, that is). During puberty, thin dark hairs begin to appear on your Venus mound and alongside your labia. Gradually, they multiply until eventually a dense, triangular meadow of hair spreads all the way back to your butt, and often spills over to your inner thighs, crossing the famous bikini line.

Aesthetic ideals of hairless or well-coiffed vulvas have become popular again in recent years—a source of anxiety and problems for many women. A lot of people worry that hair removal results in more hair, darker hair, or even causes the hairs to grow faster. For many years, we were also terrified that our bikini lines would grow uncontrollably in all directions if we weren't careful with the razor. For the same reason, many a teenage boy has regularly borrowed Dad's razor and shaved his lip fluff in the hope that a manly beard will sprout and conceal his acne. Happily for us, but unhappily for the teenage boy, this is total nonsense.

Genes and hormones determine how much body hair you get and when it grows.[30] At birth, you come equipped with all the hair follicles you'll ever have—around five million. Some of them, for example those around your sex organs and in your armpits, are especially hormone-sensitive. In puberty, our bodies explode with sex hormones, causing these follicles to enlarge and produce thicker, darker hair. The pattern for hormone-sensitive follicles varies from one person to the next depending on genes, which explains why some men have dense fur on their back while others barely have a single hair on their chest. Although it might seem like it, you don't actually get more hair in puberty; it's just that the soft down gradually transforms into "grown-up" hair. The reason a lot of people think shaving stimulates hair growth is simply that we often start to shave when our hair growth is still in the process of changing.

Some people also think that hairs become thicker and stiffer or grow more quickly when they shave. That isn't possible either, although it can feel that way when you're sitting there the day after shaving with pubes like a porcupine. Our hairs mostly consist of dead material. In fact, all the hair that is visible above the skin is dead protein and the only life to be found is down in the follicle. If you cut your hair, the follicle has no way of knowing it. The dead only speak in *Ghost Hunters*. In the real world, the follicle keeps on producing hair at exactly the same rate as before, blissfully ignorant of the fact that you are ruthlessly mowing down everything it manages to create.

The size of the follicle determines how thick the hair is. No matter how much you shave, the size of the follicle won't change. That said, hair can feel stiffer when it's shorter and starting to grow out. Normal hair that's left to its own devices wears thinner and thinner toward the tip, which is why it feels soft. When we shave, we cut the hair at its thickest point—close to the surface of the skin. So when it grows out again, the tip is thicker for a while.[31]

* * *

We may curse (or treasure) our hair growth, but the distribution of our body hair is genetically preordained. Whether you opt to do something about hair growth, however, is your choice. The hair on your body definitely has a function, but it isn't so important that you'd be better off not removing it if that's what you want to do. It is worth noting, though, that hairs help to heighten our sexual sensitivity. If your partner strokes you lightly over your pubic hair, the bending of the hairs will send a signal to the follicles, which will pass the message on to your nervous system.[32] Our follicles are connected to many nerve endings, so without hair we lose a part of the sensory experience.

Throughout history, different forms of hair removal have been normal practice for both sexes. Nowadays, you have a range of temporary solutions, including shaving, waxing, epilating, or using hair removal cream. For the most part, the choice is a matter of taste, although there are certain differences in the outcome.[33]

Epilation and waxing can lead to thinner hair growth long term, because the follicles are damaged over time when you rip hairs out by the root. The disadvantage of these methods is that thinner hairs find it harder to penetrate the skin, which can lead to problems with ingrown hairs and inflammation of the follicles. Hair removal cream "dissolves" the part of the hair that lies above the surface of the skin by destroying the hair's protein structure. Since the follicle isn't affected, people often have fewer problems with ingrown hairs when using removal creams than when they use the other methods.

There are a lot of names for the biggest problem with hair removal: razor bumps, ingrown hairs, and pseudofolliculitis barbae.[34] When you remove hair, especially if it's curly, it can turn back on itself and grow down into the skin when regrowth begins. The body registers the ingrown hair as a foreign body and this triggers an inflammation in the follicle, similar to a pimple. If you're unlucky or if you pick the bump, you could get a bacterial infection as well. Then it may become painful and swollen, and often results in scarring. In the worst-case scenario the infection may spread. It's possible to get such a serious infection in the follicle that it can grow to the size of a grape. In that case, you should consult a doctor who can gently drain the abscess and also give you a prescription if necessary.

Advice about bump-free hair removal abounds in the media. And we swallow the beauty experts' advice hook, line, and sinker—after all, a clean-shaven crotch with ingrown hairs and blemishes is hardly a pretty sight. But do you really need that $65 cream the waxing salon is trying to sell you? Or Gillette Venus ProSkin for Sensitive Skin at about $5 per blade?

Unfortunately, you're throwing your money away. If you're really bothered by ingrown hair and follicle infections, it's worth trying hair removal creams instead of the other methods. But if you do prefer epilating, waxing, or shaving, it's important to pay attention to hygiene. Wash the area well before you start. People who are prone to follicular infections would do well to rinse the area with an antibacterial toner or lotion after hair removal. These are products you can buy over the counter at the pharmacy for much less money than you'd pay for the specialized products sold in fancy bottles at salons.

THE FIVE COMMANDMENTS OF SHAVING

1. **Don't shave against the hair or stretch your skin**. When you pull your skin taut and shave against the hair, you'll get the smoothest and softest result, since you'll be cutting the hairs beneath the surface of the skin. Unfortunately, that makes it easier for the hairs to become embedded in the skin as they grow, resulting in inflammation of the follicle.

2. **Always use a clean, sharp razor blade, preferably a new one**. It's tempting to use the same razor blade many times because they're so expensive, but that's a false economy. A sharp blade cuts the hair more cleanly, allowing it to grow out more easily without getting embedded in the skin, and doesn't require you to press as hard, which helps prevent irritation and razor bumps. In addition, a used blade is covered in bacteria, which can cause follicles to become infected.

3. **Use (cheap) razor blades with a single blade**. Razor blades come in increasingly fancy versions, with an ever-growing number of blades and higher prices, usually boasting "a closer shave." Now, this may come as a surprise, but multiple blades actually result in more ingrown hairs, because each additional blade causes the hair to be cut even farther beneath the surface of the skin. What's more, the high price means that a lot of people avoid changing blades as often as they should, so that the blades become blunt and covered in bacteria. Men's razor blades are often cheaper, so it may be worth buying them instead.

4. **Use plenty of warm water**. Dry shaving should be avoided at all costs. Dry hair is stiffer and therefore harder to cut. You have to use more force, which will irritate your skin more, increasing the likelihood of red bumps and inflammation. A warm shower is an effective way of getting softer hair. Shaving foam has the same effect if you leave it on for five minutes before you shave, although it has little effect the way most people use it (quick on, quick off).

5. **Mild exfoliation**. If you're experiencing ingrown hairs, washing the area with gentle, circular movements, either with an exfoliating glove or a grainy exfoliating wash, can eventually help work them free from the skin. Don't go at it too hard, because that can lead to more irritation and skin inflammation.

DESIGNER GENITALS—WHY SOME PUT
THEIR VULVAS UNDER THE KNIFE

There's nothing new about women (and men) choosing to alter their appearance through surgery. Breast enhancements, nose jobs, liposuction, face-lifts—some people go a long way to fulfill their aesthetic ideals. However, altering your vulva through intimate surgery is a relatively new trend.

The phrase "intimate surgery" refers to all forms of surgical alteration of the external sex organs. This may involve injecting fat, smoothing out and removing fat, reducing, or expanding. A lot is possible, but the most common form of intimate surgery is labioplasty. This is plastic surgery on the labia and it's the inner labia in particular that are subject to alteration, usually to make them shorter.

We view the growing trend of intimate surgery as problematic. We're not writing this section because we look down on women who want to alter their genitals after birth, for example, or because we think that women don't have the right to decide for themselves what to do with their bodies. Of course, you should decide for yourself—this is about something else. We're writing about this topic because we're afraid a group of young women are opting for intimate surgery on the basis of a misunderstanding. In our experience, many women with normal, healthy genitals are choosing intimate surgery because they think there's something wrong with their body. This misunderstanding needs to be corrected and to do that we have to go back to anatomy.

We make a distinction between medical and aesthetic reasons for choosing labioplasty. There's a difference between wanting to have a nose job because you have difficulty breathing through your nose and because you don't like the way your nose looks. In the same way, there's a difference between trimming your labia because you're struggling with pain or difficulty having intercourse and because you don't think your genitals look nice. The length of your inner labia is only a medical issue if they cause you problems.

This doesn't necessarily mean that there's anything wrong with wanting to have surgery for aesthetic reasons, but if you are going to choose to take this step it's important that the choice you make is based on knowledge, not misunderstandings.

Many women think their inner labia should always be hidden, entirely packed away inside the outer labia, but it's normal for the inner labia of adult women to protrude a long way beyond their outer labia. In fact, there's no one way women are supposed to look down there. What we do have in common is the various parts that combine to form our vulva: the inner and outer labia, the clitoris, the urinary opening, and the vaginal opening. But these parts look different from one woman to the next; there is an unbelievable amount of variation. Even so the belief that the inner labia should be short and hidden is surprisingly strong among many women. In an Australian study that interviewed women between eighteen and twenty-eight, all the women picked out an image of a hairless vulva with concealed inner labia when they were asked what society's "ideal vulva" was.[35]

Where, precisely, does this idea come from, since there are so many wonderful, varied genitals? As with other forms of body image pressure, we might consider the ideals of popular culture, pornography, and so on. They're certainly part of the problem, at least. The difficulty when it comes to aesthetic ideals about the vulva in particular is that it's harder to confirm whether these are rooted in reality. Once a person has established a belief that normal genitals have short labia, this belief will be stronger than the idea that normal hair is all straight. After all, we see people's hairstyles all day, every day; we know that they come in all textures and lengths so it's easy to knock down that idea. However, we don't often see other women's genitals except during an intimate moment, especially as communal showers become more unpopular and people are uncomfortable being seen naked. Being naked is no longer natural. Being naked is all too often about sex, and, for many women, displaying their bodies is connected with shame.

We believe the misunderstanding surrounding the inner labia arises in part because of a critical gap in school curriculum when it comes to pubertal development. Like the rest of the body, female genitals change a great deal in puberty, but we cannot personally remember having been told at any time exactly what happens to the genitals in puberty. At school we heard about how the penis grows, we heard about how breasts grow, and we heard about the different parts of the body that gradually become covered in hair. We learned an awful lot, but we didn't learn what happens to the inner labia when we pass from childhood to adulthood.

The fact is that most female children have genitals whose outer labia cover their inner labia. In other words, we all become familiar with and accustomed to genitals that are formed in this way when we are children. But in puberty the inner labia begin to grow. For many women, they become so long that they protrude a good way beyond the outer labia, and they often become folded, crinkled, and uneven in terms of thickness.

If you've always had genitals whose outer labia cover their inner labia, it can come as a shock if this suddenly changes, especially if nobody's warned you that it's going to happen and that it's normal. The feeling that something is wrong can be reinforced if you ask friends about it and they happen not to have visible inner labia. After all, both types are common.

In other words, some women believe the only normal or "correct" genitals are the ones shaped like those we have as children. If young women had learned as early as elementary school that their genitals would change, and if they'd gotten to know more about what they might look like between the legs once they were adults, perhaps we wouldn't have seen this recent increase in intimate surgery. We could at least have eliminated the misunderstandings that lead some women to go undergo surgery.

It's important to remember what the inner labia do (they have a sexual function) and what it can mean to trim them. They're full of nerve endings and it feels good to touch them. When you cut your labia, you're removing an important and sensitive part of your genitals, and, as always, operations involve risk. In the worst case, it's possible there will be scar tissue that may be unsightly and cause permanent pain, and that's why you should always think carefully before undergoing an operation to alter your labia.

INTERNAL SEX ORGANS—THE HIDDEN TREASURES

It can be easy to forget that the female sex organs are much more than just the vulva and vagina, but beneath the layers of skin, fat, and muscle lies a set of soft, hidden body parts that include the internal sex organs.

Let's start the journey in. If you stick a finger into your vagina, you'll feel a soft little projection about seven to ten centimeters in, with the same consistency and shape as the tip of your nose—just a little bigger. That's the cervix: the entrance to the uterus. From the vagina, the cervix looks sort of like a flattened sphere. At first glance, it doesn't appear to have an exit or entrance, but right in the middle it actually has a tiny little hole called the mouth of the uterus. This is the start of an extremely narrow passage two to three centimeters in length that leads us to the uterus's interior. It is through this thin passage that the menstrual fluids, as well as discharge, seep out. In fact, this small passageway is where most discharge is produced.

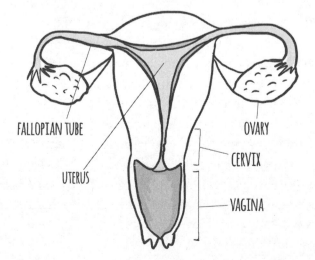

FALLOPIAN TUBE

OVARY

CERVIX

UTERUS

VAGINA

Many people think the passage from the vagina to the uterus is wide open. We've often been asked the following question: If you have sex when you're pregnant is it possible for the penis to hit the baby? There are a lot of people who wonder about sex and the uterus. If you've read the Murakami novel *Kafka on the Shore*, you probably enjoyed the paragraph where a woman felt a man's sperm spraying against the walls of her uterus,[36] as if the penis were inside the woman's uterus when the man ejaculated. You can't get a penis into a uterus (even if the sperm can eventually make its way up there—that is kind of the point). The cervix isn't an open airlock; it's closed. In any case, the vagina is more than deep enough to accommodate most penises, thanks to its elasticity. It simply isn't necessary to go farther in.

Our impression has been that most women aren't aware of their own cervix, which isn't really so surprising. But the cervix actually deserves all the attention you can give it, for the sake of your health. The cervix is a part of the body where young women can be struck by cancer. In addition, it is often the place where many of the symptoms of sexually transmitted disease manifest themselves.

However important it is, the cervix is just a small part of a larger organ, the womb or *uterus*. The uterus is normally a small organ the size of a fist, but if you're pregnant it expands dramatically. After all, it needs to become big enough to carry one (or more) growing embryos to term. In premenopausal adult women, the uterus is around 7.5 centimeters long and weighs no more than 2.5 ounces. The uterus most resembles an upside-down pear, with the cervix as the narrow part that the stalk grows out of.

Most women's uteruses are tipped forward, toward their navel, so that they're at a roughly 90-degree angle to the vagina. That's one more reason why a penis can never get into the uterus: it can't bend when it's erect, because if it did, it would break. The penis is no contortionist! Twenty percent of all women have a backward-leaning uterus, which works just as well as a forward-leaning one. It's a bit like the way some people have blue eyes and others have brown: You can still see just the same.

The uterus is hollow, but not in the same way that a barrel is hollow, because it doesn't contain air. The uterus's anterior and posterior walls are pressed tightly up against each other, just like the vaginal walls. Between them lies a thin layer of fluid.

The uterus has very thick muscular walls. These muscles are necessary when, for example, clotted menstrual fluid needs to be pushed out through the extremely narrow passage in the cervix. The muscles in the uterus contract then, like a dishcloth being wrung out. When you get menstrual pains, it feels as if you're having cramps in your stomach or your back, but the pains actually come from the uterus itself, as it works to push out the blood and mucus.

The wall of the uterus has several layers, and the innermost layer, the endometrium, is a mucous membrane. It changes enormously over the course of the menstrual cycle and plays a central role in menstruation. It grows large and thick every month and if you don't become pregnant, it's expelled from the uterus. It's worth remembering the name "endometrium" because it's related to a condition that bothers an awful lot of women: *endometriosis*. This is a disease in which the uterine lining grows in other areas of the body in addition to the inside of the uterus. Among other effects, this condition is responsible for extra-painful periods. You'll learn more about endometriosis later on in the book (pages 204–8).

Think of the uterus as a triangle, with one corner pointing downward and two thin tubes projecting from each of the upper corners. Known as the fallopian tubes, they extend about ten centimeters to either side and their purpose is to carry the egg from the ovaries down to the uterus. At the end of each tube are small finger-like projections called *fimbriae*, which stretch out toward the ovaries to catch the eggs they release. Fertilization of the egg by the sperm takes place in the fallopian tube, and the fertilized egg then floats into the uterus, where it fastens itself to the endometrium in order to grow.

The ovaries are like small bags or sacks. We have two of them, one on either side of the uterus, and they have two tasks. The first is to develop and store the eggs, which are the woman's sex cells. Unlike men, women don't produce new sex cells over the course of their life. We are born with about 300,000 eggs.[37] But these eggs are not yet mature. The ones we have at birth are actually just precursors of fertile eggs. These pre-eggs are already formed by the fifth month of an embryo's life. Up until puberty, when the menstrual cycle starts up, these pre-eggs will rehearse for their future task. They begin to mature in batches, but since they don't receive the ovulation signal from the brain, they simply end up dying. In massive numbers. By the time we reach puberty, we've lost over a third of our eggs to these practice runs and are left with an exclusive group of around 180,000 eggs. By the time we're twenty-five, we have approximately 65,000 left. These eggs must patiently await their turn, and will mature and be released one menstrual cycle after another.

Now perhaps you're thinking it's peculiar that we have 180,000 eggs at the start of puberty. We're obviously not going to have periods that many times over the course of our lives, so what are we doing with tens of thousands of eggs? The truth—and this came as a surprise to us as well—is that we can actually use up to a thousand eggs every single month, not just one, as is commonly described. The number used each month varies throughout our life and slows down significantly the older we get. That's how the numbers add up, if you tried to do the math.

In other words, the difference between our eggs and a man's sperm isn't as vast as it's often made out to be. For women, as for men, multiple sex cells fight a hard battle among themselves for the right to try and make a baby. A battalion of eggs begin to mature every month, but only one select egg makes it through security and is released from the ovary. The rest are brutally rejected and destroyed.[38]

Several times, we've come up against an interesting question about hormonal contraception: Will contraception that prevents ovulation make your eggs and fertility last longer? After all, it sounds logical that it would be worth the body's while to save the eggs until you were ready to make a baby instead disposing of them every month through menstruation. Unfortunately it doesn't work that way. Hormonal contraception only prevents that single, chosen egg from being released from the ovary each month; it doesn't prevent the monthly maturation of a thousand pre-eggs. You'll lose just as many eggs each month, no matter how much contraception you use.[39]

Between the ages of about forty-five to fifty-five[40] we normally reach menopause, a phase of life in which the female body undergoes just as many dramatic changes as it did in puberty. The most important change is that we cease to be fertile. We have simply used up our egg reserves. The age of menopause varies from one woman to the next and its timing is largely determined by genetics. What's more, some women naturally have more eggs than others. However, men continue to produce sperm cells until the moment their hearts stop beating—up to several million a day. Their fertility has no best-before date, although the sperm often diminishes in quality over the years.[*] Mick Jagger became a father for the eighth time in 2016 at the age of seventy-three, with his much younger ballerina girlfriend. Sometimes the world is unfair.

The ovaries' second task is to produce hormones. The most important and best known of these are estrogen and progesterone. These hormones alter our bodies throughout our various phases of life, and they control the menstrual cycle in collaboration with several other hormones from different areas, including the brain. But we'll come back to that later.

GENDER, GENDER, AND GENDER

For many people, the word *gender* contains an opposition: woman/man, girl/boy. You may hear the question "What is a man?" or "What is a woman?" and think it's easy to answer: Of course a man

---

[*]   In other words, the man's age influences the couple's fertility and the child's risk of congenital disease.

is a person with a man's body, and a woman is a person with a woman's body. *The Wonder Down Under*, for example, is a book about people who have a vagina and other female sex organs, so that must mean it's a book about women, right?

It's hardly surprising you might think this way, but it's not actually that simple. Whether we are women or men is not determined only by our sex organs or our body shape. What's more, the physical difference between the sexes is much smaller than you think.

In this section, we'll focus on three factors that are involved in determining just what gender we are: our chromosomes, which we refer to here as *genetic gender*; our bodies, or *physical gender*; and psychological factors, or *psychological gender*. We are not saying that these are the only factors that constitute "gender." We could also talk about social and cultural factors, of course. But since this is a medical book, we've opted to focus on the genetic, physical, and psychological.

GENETIC GENDER—A COOKBOOK

Have you ever seen a picture of a DNA strand? If you zoom in with a gigantic microscope, it looks like a ladder that's been twisted into a spiral. But the rungs on the DNA ladder aren't like the ones on the stepladder you use when you're changing a lightbulb. In relation to its width, which is less than microscopic, the DNA ladder is insanely tall and has very special rungs.

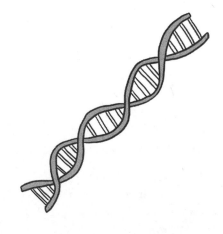

The rungs are made of substances that we can compare to letters. On each rung there are two letters. Together, they can be read as codes or small recipes. Each recipe encodes a protein that carries out a specific task in the body. When they're put together, we call the codes for several proteins a *gene*. Our genes determine whether we have blue or brown eyes, two or three legs, wings and tails, or big brains. In conjunction, all these codes are a bit like a cookbook filled with recipes for absolutely every component we need to make *us* specifically. The fancy name for this kind of cookbook is a *genome*. Our genome is our entire genetic recipe.

Every single cell in the body contains a complete genome (or cookbook) for the person the cell comes from, meaning that there are around ten feet of DNA strands in every cell. This is what the police rely on when they use blood, sperm, nails, or skin cells to look for criminals. If you take a totally random cell from another person, for example the one and only Queen B, Beyoncé, this cell will, in theory, contain all the information you need to build a new version of her—in other words, a clone. But how can an entire ten-foot cookbook fit into something as small as a cell? Well, the long DNA strands are coiled into densely packed bundles, just like a ball of yarn, so that everything can fit. Within each cell we have forty-six such bundles, which combine to constitute the whole genetic code, i.e., the entire cookbook. These bundles are known as chromosomes.

The chromosomes are organized into pairs. So we have forty-six chromosomes in twenty-three pairs, and within each pair, one bundle comes from our mother and one from our father.

When it comes to gender, there's only one pair of chromosomes that counts: the twenty-third, which are our sex chromosomes. These two bundles are the ones that determine whether we are male or female, genetically speaking. There are two types of sex chromosome, known as X and Y. Females have two chromosomes of the same type, coded XX, while males have one X variant and one Y variant, coded XY.

As you may recall, we started off with one cell from the mother (the egg cell) and one from the father (the sperm cell). Each cell contains half a set of each chromosome, i.e., twenty-three single bundles, or half a cookbook. When you make a baby, you put together half a cookbook from the mother and half a cookbook from the father, giving the child a whole cookbook containing a recipe that is unique in its composition.

Since people who are genetically female never have a Y chromosome, just two Xs, an egg cell will always contain an X version of the sex chromosome. This is the mother's contribution to the embryo's twenty-third chromosome pair. The mother will never be able to offer a Y. However, the father's sex cell, the sperm cell, may contain either an X or a Y. Around half of sperm cells contain an X and the other half a Y. If a sperm cell containing a Y combines with the egg, the embryo will be male, because the code is XY. If a sperm cell containing an X combines with the egg, the embryo will be female, coded XX.

As such, it is always the man who "decides" whether the child will be a genetic male or female. Historically there has been a great deal of pressure on women to "give men sons." You may have read about this in relation to frustrated kings waiting for their queen to produce a suitable heir, who must *of course* be a man.

These days we know better. It's pure chance whether the child is male or female; there's a fifty-fifty chance every time,* depending on which sperm cell from the man combines with the egg. The woman's egg cell has no influence over the child's sex.

What we can conclude from all this is the following: If the twenty-third chromosome pair contains two X chromosomes, the embryo's cookbook says: "to be developed into a female." If the twenty-third chromosome pair contains both types of chromosome, X and Y, the cookbook says: "to be developed into a male."

This all seems nice and easy, and with these recipes in mind you may get the impression that gender is just a matter of "either/or." But, as you'll soon see, that's far from the case. In fact, as we've mentioned previously, men's and women's sex organs are incredibly

---

*   Actually it isn't exactly fifty-fifty. For one reason or another, slightly more boys than girls are born when nature gets her way.

similar, and many in-between things can come about in the process of reaching a finished sex organ. We often tend to focus a bit too hard on the differences, but after all, we have more between our legs than just "a hole or a stick."

It's also true that one thing or another can go awry, both with the chromosomes and the individual genes in the DNA, and as a result the recipe can come out not quite as expected. And a mix-up in a recipe means that the result will also be different—it's a bit like adding a cup of oil instead of a cup of butter. It may still taste good, but it's definitely different from what you'd pictured.

In fact, people can be born with too many or too few sex chromosomes; what gender does that make them? What gender is X, XXX, or XXY? That's a good question. (As you've probably realized by now, there's no such thing as YY, because it's impossible for two sperm cells to make a baby together.)

To get to the bottom of all this, we need to talk a bit about how our sex organs develop, which makes this a good moment to introduce the second aspect of gender: *physical gender*.

PHYSICAL GENDER—BODY AND SEX ORGANS

So far, we've seen that the egg cell and the sperm cell combine and, if nothing goes amiss, we're left with an XX or an XY recipe—i.e., *female* or *male*. In spite of that, the male and female embryos are no different from each other at the start. In the beginning, the embryos are *absolutely identical* regardless of their chromosome combination. An embryo always starts off with gender-neutral genitalia, which have the potential to become either (or both) female and male sex organs, and the embryo's internal sex organs can just as easily become testicles as ovaries.

For simplicity's sake, we'll focus mostly on the external sex organs here. Turn the page to see how they look right at the beginning.

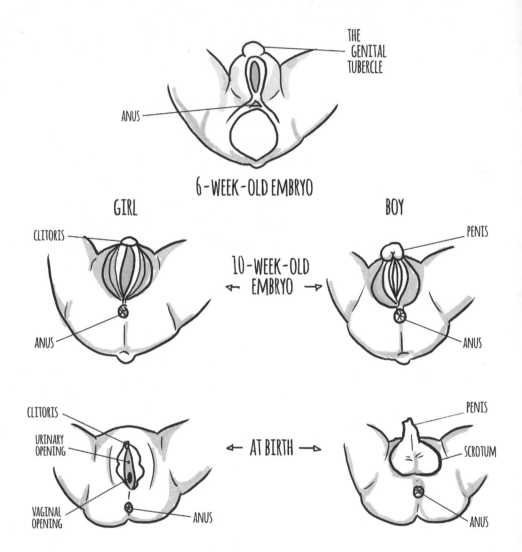

THE
GENITAL
TUBERCLE

ANUS

6-WEEK-OLD EMBRYO

GIRL   BOY

CLITORIS   PENIS

10-WEEK-OLD
← EMBRYO →

ANUS   ANUS

CLITORIS   PENIS

URINARY
OPENING   ← AT BIRTH →   SCROTUM

VAGINAL
OPENING   ANUS

ANUS

Uppermost in the genital area lies the genital tubercle. It looks a bit like a mini-penis, doesn't it, or perhaps a clitoris? The genital tubercle actually has the ability to become either.

In order for the gender-neutral embryonic genitalia to develop into male sex organs, the embryo needs everything to go according to a precise plan over the course of a few critical days pretty early in the pregnancy. The embryo must in fact be influenced by male sex hormones at precisely the right time. The most important hormone in this game is testosterone, which is only produced if the embryo has a Y chromosome. If an embryo with a Y chromosome isn't influenced by testosterone, most often because of a genetic error in one or more of the male embryo's genes, the genital area automatically forms into a vulva. That results in a *genetic* male who has the sex organs of a female.

In other words, the vulva is what all embryos come equipped with unless a special counter-command is issued. Some men have taken this to mean that men "have something extra," whereas women are more basic—a white T-shirt compared with a fancy party top, say, although you can interpret it as you wish. You could just as easily say that women are the primary and fundamental sex, whereas men are a variant, the second sex. But, hang on a minute . . . wasn't that used to describe women?

Look at the illustration of gender development on page 36. As we said earlier, the little knob at the top of the embryo's genital area, the genital tubercle, can become either a penis or a clitoris. If you know a bit about the penis and if you read the section about the clitoris earlier in the book (pages 8–11), you'll realize that the two have a lot in common.

This is particularly important for women who are stressed out by the size of their clitoral glans. We're fed the idea that the clitoris is supposed to be like a sweet little button; however, your outer parts may well stick out a long way. That doesn't mean you're more like a man! Clitorises come in different sizes, just like penises, which can be anything from 7 to 20 centimeters (about 2.5 to 8 inches) long. A shorter penis doesn't make a man a woman.

But back to our embryo: The male urethra fuses with the penis, while the female urethra becomes a separate unit. Folds form on either side of the growing clitoris-penis. These become either the male *scrotum* or the *labia majora* (the outer labia). For the folds to become a scrotum, they must fuse together in the middle. To become labia, they do not fuse, but just grow a little.

If you don't believe us when we say that a man's external genitalia are very much like our own, you should take a good look between the legs of the next man you see naked. As you'll see, his scrotum is divided in two by a neat, thin line, just like a seam. And guess what—it *is* a seam! This is where the labia have fused together to become a scrotum! The penis is nothing but an overgrown clitoris with an inbuilt urethra: imagine shrinking it massively, shifting the urethra a bit farther down and dividing the scrotum in two, and you'll get a kind of vulva.

Wow! That's pretty cool, but don't go cutting up your boyfriend or any other men you happen to meet. Men need their scrotums to keep their testicles in. Having said that, this is pretty much what surgeons do when they perform gender confirmation surgery from a male to a female body, but we'll come back to *that* later.

Returning to the question of chromosomal irregularities, all embryos without a Y chromosome become physically female, while all those with a Y chromosome are influenced by testosterone so that the fetus becomes physically male. Or wiped out, according to the popular postapocalyptic comic book series, *Y: The Last Man*. No, we are just pulling your leg.

These are theoretical cases, but if a given fetus is coded X or XXX, its cookbook will say it's female. If it has Y or XXY coding, the recipe will point toward male development. But as in other cookbooks, the result isn't always as described in the recipe. It is possible to develop into a woman, physically speaking, even if you are genetically a man—and vice versa!

Some fetuses that are genetically male may have difficulty responding to the testosterone produced in the body. In the absence of testosterone, they'll become female on the outside, with a vulva between their legs instead of a penis and scrotum. Varying gradations of this condition exist. Some people may be born without a uterus and with testicles between their legs rather than ovaries in their belly, even though they have a vulva. It's also possible to end up with external genitalia that have developed to a point somewhere in between the penis-balls complex (male sex organs) and the vulva.

There are children born every year who cause the midwife to scratch her head when the parents ask if it's a boy or a girl. The fact is, it's not certain the midwife will be able to give them an answer. These types of diagnoses may be called intersex,* which simply means "in-between sex." Disorders of sex development, or "DSD," is also a commonly used term.

The case we described earlier, in which there is no correspondence between the genetic gender and the outer sex organs, is also a type of intersexuality. As you see, intersexuality can take many forms. It may be that external genitalia do not match a gender, or that the external and internal genitalia correspond to different genders or both genders.

Many children who are born with intersex traits are operated on, which brings us to a sad history lesson. Until the 1990s, all children who were born with "ambiguous" external genitalia were surgically assigned female. At the time, people thought this would be fine since gender was seen as being dependent on socialization. As long as you brought the child up in a given gender, it would feel itself to be that gender. If a child was given dolls and pink clothes, many people believed that would do the trick.

Surgeons also thought it was easier to achieve a successful outcome if they made a vulva rather than a penis and balls. The surgeons, who were usually men themselves, felt that a person couldn't

* There are many views about the term intersex. It may be used to describe a group of medical conditions, or an identity. We think it's a good term for describing physical variants between male and female development, but we're aware that different people prefer different terms when they are talking about themselves.

have a good life with a small, only semi-functional penis, whereas a semi-functional vulva wouldn't be a problem for women. After all, sex was more important for men. The result was that they made *physical* girls out of children who, *genetically* and *psychologically*, were boys. Many lives have been ruined this way.

The increasingly widespread acknowledgment of the harmful mental side effects of this custom has caused many surgeons to change their practice dramatically. These doctors now encourage parents to delay surgery and prefer to do more in-depth examinations to determine gender, so that hopefully the child will end up with a body that is the "right gender" after an operation. They no longer operate on the baby immediately after birth, but often take several years to examine the child instead.

There has been some debate around this kind of treatment. Many people think these children shouldn't be operated on at all, but should be allowed to decide for themselves what they want to do once they reach adulthood. The people who take this view think the entire idea that everybody must fit into the "boy" or "girl" mold is wrong in principle. Why isn't it acceptable to be something in between? Why can't we just bring up children as "they" and let them discover their own sexual identity over time? This brings us to the third aspect of gender: psychological gender.

PSYCHOLOGICAL GENDER—A QUESTION OF IDENTITY

Psychological gender is more difficult to explain through biology, because our psychological gender is a question of identity: how we think about ourselves and who we are. This is personal, and only you can know what is right for you.

Many important things are overlooked because we think far too much about what is "normal." For most people, the three factors all point toward one gender. We feel as if we're women, we look like women between our legs, and our genes confirm that we are female. But the fact that most of us experience things one way doesn't mean it's the same for *everybody*—a lesson humanity is constantly having to learn over and over again.

When your son says he's a girl, only wants to wear dresses, and prefers his big sister's Barbie collection to a train set and football, it's easy to insist that it's just a phase, but that isn't necessarily true. Nor is it a given that people must be "feminine" or prefer dolls to sports in order to be girls. Psychological gender is not the same as personality and need not be based on traditional gender roles. Nonetheless, it is quite possible for people's psychological gender to differ from their genital and genetic gender. We often use the terms *trans* or "born in the wrong body" to describe people with a gender different from the one indicated by their bodies and their genes.

So what does it mean to be trans? The word *trans* comes from Latin, meaning "through," "to cross," or "to change," as in "to transcend." The term *trans* is used for a person who identifies as a gender different than the one he or she belongs to genetically or physically. People may also call themselves trans if they don't identify with a specific gender; not everybody feels the need for that kind of specific label. *Trans* is often marked with an asterisk: *trans**. This is done to show that *trans* is a broad term encompassing many things. It may, for example, be worth asking a transperson what pronouns they prefer: he, she, they, or something else entirely? You won't necessarily know in advance, so ask if you're wondering—it's better than just making an assumption and potentially embarrassing yourself or making someone else feel uncomfortable.

People who aren't trans are called *cis*. This also comes from Latin and means the opposite of "to cross." *Cis* is a word that implies "staying on this side of something."

A transwoman is a person who was born in a male body but is nonetheless a woman, and who may wish to change her body so that her physical and psychological genders match. A transman is a person who was born in a female body, but identifies as a man.

Many trans people know from childhood that they belong to a gender that doesn't match their body. This may seem terrifying to many parents, in the same way that other unknown things seem terrifying. So it's important for us to talk about transgender issues and raise awareness about them. If people suspect their child has been "born in the wrong body," the child can be referred to a specialist by the family's pediatrician. If appropriate, the child can eventually be given gender confirmation treatment, with the help of hormones and operations.

Fortunately, people are becoming more used to the concept of being trans, generally through popular culture. The actress Laverne Cox of Netflix's *Orange Is the New Black* and Caitlyn Jenner, of Kardashian family fame, are among those who have put transgender issues on the map in recent years. In Norway, the series *Born in the Wrong Body* has attracted a lot of attention (there was a short-lived British and American version in 2007; perhaps it would last longer these days). Americans are probably quite familiar with the former soldier Chelsea Manning, who was infamously convicted of espionage under her birth name, Bradley Manning, after giving classified information to WikiLeaks, and with Laura Jane Grace, the lead singer of punk band Against Me!, who came out as a transwoman to *Rolling Stone* in 2012 and has since become a trans advocate and icon.

There are (at least) three factors that determine which gender we belong to; the ones we discussed here are genetic, physical, and psychological gender. Remember, gender need not be binary. We may have chromosomal errors that mean we don't have the typical chromosome combination of XX or XY. We may have genetic irregularities that have formed us into something in between woman and man during the physical development of our sex organs. It is also possible for your psychological gender to differ from the genital and genetic gender you were born with. In other words, gender isn't as simple as it might seem. We hope this overview has sparked your curiosity and made you a little more open to the mosaic of possibilities that gender presents.

PART 2: DISCHARGE, PERIODS, AND OTHER GORE

Like the other orifices in our bodies, the vagina is an exit and not just an entrance. Out of it comes screaming babies, blood, mucus, and gore. This makes it a source of immense joy as well as embarrassment, and some of it gives us ways of finding out if there's anything wrong down there. And then there are the hormones—the signal substances that run the whole show. The time has come to talk about the slightly less tangible parts of our sexual apparatus.

DOUCHEBAGS AND DISCO MICE

Discharge. Let the word roll around on your tongue. It's an odd word that calls to mind plumbing systems and sewage pipes. Discharge is most familiar to us as the slick, milky, or yellowish-white stain that makes a regular appearance in our underwear after puberty. It's what makes our underwear dirty. Perhaps it's hardly surprising discharge isn't a hot topic or something we tend to discuss at top volume. But what actually is discharge? Is there any difference between different types of moisture down there? And why should we bother thinking about discharge in the first place?

Let's get one thing straight right away: All healthy girls who've reached puberty will find discharge in their underwear. Every single day. It's a fluid that seeps out of our vaginas continuously from the very first day our sexual organs come under the influence of a hormone called estrogen at the onset of puberty. Some of the discharge comes from glands in the cervix. As mentioned earlier, the vagina itself doesn't have any glands, but a lot of fluid seeps through the walls of the vagina, mingling with fluid from the cervix and from the glands at the opening of the vagina, including Bartholin's glands.

Normally, between a half and a whole teaspoonful of discharge will seep out over the course of a day, although this varies depending on the individual woman as well as the point she is at in her cycle and her vaginal health.[1] Some women who use hormonal contraception find that their discharge levels increase, as do pregnant women. The consistency of the discharge will also vary, ranging from a runny liquid to a slimy, thread-like substance similar to egg whites just before ovulation.

Discharge isn't just normal—it's necessary. It turns the vagina into a self-cleaning tube. The purpose of the discharge is to keep the vagina clean and to flush out unwelcome guests such as fungi and bacteria, as well as dead cells from the surface of the mucous membrane. In addition, it usually contains masses of good lactic acid bacteria, known as lactobacilli. These produce—yes, you've guessed it—lactic acid, which is what gives the discharge its slightly acidic taste and smell.

Even more important, the lactic acids create the low pH that is absolutely essential to a healthy vagina. Most of the bacteria that cause disease don't thrive in an acidic environment. In addition, all the lactic acid bacteria prevent potentially harmful bacteria from finding the conditions they need to grow, because they're all competing for the same space and the same nutrition. The end result is that infections are prevented. In short, discharge keeps our vaginas healthy.

At the same time, it lubricates the mucous membranes and keeps them moist. Dry mucous membranes are easily torn and once that happens, problems quickly follow. Just think what your mouth would be like without spit. Without discharge, the mucous membranes in the vagina tear and you can get little sores. Sex becomes a nightmare and the likelihood of sexually transmitted infections also increases because the body's outer barrier has been damaged. In other words, discharge isn't some dirty thing that should be flushed out of our vaginas, but an important ally.

The problem is that people think it's icky—as if discharge were a sign of being dirty or having poor hygiene. Very few girls will leave their used underwear lying around or hanging out in the bathroom. In some environments, things have gone so far that people think the vagina itself should be flushed clean of discharge. Perhaps you've never thought about where the insult "douchebag" comes from. Nor had Nina until she moved to the United States, bought herself a bottle of intimate wash at the drugstore, and left it in the communal shower room in the dorms. After a while, a sniggering fellow student told her she should remove it because the rumors were already flying around about the Norwegian girl with the douchebag.

"Douchebag?" said Nina, a bit confused. She was quickly informed that *everybody* believed she was squirting perfumed soapy water into her vagina using a kind of bulb syringe—apparently common practice among sex workers and many other women. Nina tried to explain that it was just regular vaginal wash, pH 3.5 and all that, but she quickly gave up trying to convince her fellow students. "Nice girls" must never, for God's sake, draw attention to the fact that their genitals need the occasional wash. Even admitting that you washed your genitals was taboo, as if it might give away the great secret of discharge. Nina continued to leave the bottle in the showers.

Our genitals are happiest if you clean it with just warm water, an oil, or a mild intimate soap. You should never use ordinary soap on them because it can easily cause your vulnerable mucous membranes to dry out or become irritated. Itching and burning down below are often caused by using products that are too strong, or simply by washing too much. At any rate, you should never flush out your vagina, because it may actually increase the likelihood of infections.

What reason could women have for feeling they need to flush out their vaginas? For many, it's probably to do with smell. A lot of women we've spoken to are anxious about whether they smell "normal" down there. They describe worrying about whether colleagues can detect the smell of their vaginas when they're sitting side by side at a meeting, or refusing to let their sex partners go down on them in case they find their scent a turnoff.

Healthy genitals smell. That's just the way it is. Fresh discharge has a mildly acidic scent and taste because it contains lactic acid. What's more, our vulva and groin are amply equipped with sweat glands. Tight pants or shorts, underwear made of synthetic fabric, and crossed legs create a warm environment between our legs. Therefore, over the course of a long day, you will, naturally enough, sweat a great deal there. The combination of an entire day's worth of discharge and sweat together with a dash of residual urine creates a characteristic odor. In our circle of female friends, we use the Norwegian term *discomus*, meaning "disco mouse." This describes the distinctive smell your genitals—your "mouse"—give off after a long night on the dance floor, or a trip to the gym, for that matter. It doesn't exactly smell bad, but it certainly can smell pretty intense.

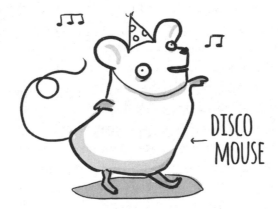

← DISCO MOUSE

The smell and quantity of discharge varies according to what phase you're at in your menstrual cycle. Our sex hormones seem to influence our body's ability to rid itself of a malodorous substance called trimethylamine, which is what can cause that classic stink of rotten fish. It has been observed that, among healthy woman, the body has 60 to 70 percent less capacity to rid itself of this substance just before and during menstruation.[2] That could explain why even healthy women may find their genitals give off a fishy smell around the time of their period.

The scent of our genitals is one of our most intimate odors. It's completely normal for them to smell a bit, especially at the end of a long day; but as a rule, they shouldn't smell bad, if you get what we mean. A bad smell may be a sign of infection and it's a good reason to pay a visit to your doctor. If you've gone for a checkup and your odor problems aren't caused by an infection, it may be a good idea to wear loose pants or skirts, change your underwear over the course of the day, and take proper (but not excessive!) care of your hygiene.

As you'll have realized, discharge is closely associated with the well-being of your sex organs, so it's hardly surprising that, with a little observation, it can tell us a lot about the situation down under. Discharge can change as a result of both infections and imbalances in the vaginal flora, but substantial changes also occur during a normal menstrual cycle.

In other words, it's important to get to know what your normal discharge is like—in terms of odor, color, and consistency. Some people produce only a little discharge while others produce such large quantities that they have to change their underwear during the day. Both can be normal. The most important thing is to know what is typical for you personally. That way, not only will you be able to work out when there's something wrong or when it's time for a trip to the doctor, but you'll also get an idea of where you are in your menstrual cycle. To give you some assistance, we've put together a discharge guide (page 48).

PERIODS—HOW TO BLEED WITHOUT DYING

It comes roughly every month. Sometimes it's painful, sometimes it's embarrassing and takes you by surprise, but most of the time everything goes smoothly. Although we could manage quite happily without vaginal bleeding each month, menstruation can be a huge relief in certain situations: *Phew—you aren't pregnant!*

DISCHARGE YOU SHOULD CHECK WITH A DOCTOR

- A copious runny discharge that is grayish-white with a fishy smell can be a sign of bacterial vaginosis, which is an imbalance in the normal vaginal flora.

- A thick, lumpy, white discharge with a normal odor may be a sign of a yeast infection.

- An increased flow of discharge, generally yellowish-white in color, may indicate infections such as chlamydia, mycoplasma, or gonorrhea. The last of these more often produces a yellowish-green discharge than the first two.

- Copious amounts of runny, foaming discharge that is yellowish-green in color and nasty smelling may be a sign of a trichomoniasis, which about 3 percent of American women ages fourteen to forty-nine will experience at some point in their lives, many—about 85 percent—without any symptoms.[3]*

- Copious amounts of whitish, possibly grainy discharge with a normal smell may be a sign of overproduction of lactobacilli, especially if you also have itching and groin pain.

- Discharge mixed with blood when not on your period—everything from small brown spots to pink, dark, or fresh blood in the discharge—may be caused by a sexually transmitted infection or abnormal cells in the cervix. You should always get any unexplained bleeding checked by a doctor.

NORMAL CHANGES IN DISCHARGE THAT ARE NO CAUSE FOR CONCERN

- Slimy egg white that you can stretch between your fingers means ovulation is imminent.

- Increased amounts of discharge with the same odor, color, and consistency as you usually have—hormonal contraception or pregnancy may be the cause.

---

* Trichomonas vaginalis is a little parasite that causes trichomoniasis. This disease is rare in Norway, but is one of the most common sexually transmitted diseases worldwide (around 3 percent of women in the United States will get it). Some people may suffer intense itching of the vulva and vagina, as well as nasty-smelling discharge and a burning sensation when peeing, while others don't notice a thing. The infection is not dangerous and is treated with metronidazole, a special type of antibiotic.

Menstruation takes up a large share of our lives. If you bleed once a month and your period lasts five days each time, you'll have up to sixty days of bleeding each year. If you have periods for forty years, that means you'll have 2,400 days of menstruation over the course of your life—equivalent to over six-and-a-half years of periods! We ought to talk a lot more about this bleeding, especially since it can involve a bunch of crappy challenges like PMS (premenstrual syndrome, which we cover on pages 60–3), uncomfortable situations, and severe pain.

These challenges may be bad enough, although the problems many women face these days are minimal compared with the troubles of our sisters in days gone by, before humans invented tampons, the menstrual cup, sanitary pads, and painkillers. In the past in some cultures, women would crochet or knit cotton sanitary pads, which had to be boiled and hung out to dry after every use. Menstruation is still a major challenge around the world. PMS fades into insignificance when you hear about girls having to give up school because of their monthly bleeding, or women who use dirty cloths and get infections because they don't have access to the clean, disposable products that are taken for granted in other parts of the world. Menstruation is frequently overlooked as a barrier to genuine equality for the women of the world. Think about that next time you're in the store buying your tampons.

Now let's focus on the bleeding itself. Most of us know that our periods are connected to fertility. Menstruation demonstrates that you have an internal cycle and that your body has the capacity to bear a child. But what is it that's actually bleeding, and where is the wound? Why does the color of menstrual blood change from brown to red, and why is it lumpy?

The blood comes because the womb, or uterus, was ready to receive a fertilized egg and didn't this time around. The uterus readies itself for pregnancy by increasing the amount of endometrium or mucous membrane—in other words the inner wall, or lining, of the uterus. The fertilized egg attaches itself to this lining, which is what will nourish the tiny growing creature by supplying it with the mother's blood. If no egg arrives, the body has no need for the thick layer of mucous membrane, so it's all expelled and bleeds away. This is what causes the slimy consistency of period blood. Some of the lumps are simply scraps of the discarded mucous membrane; the flow is not fresh blood from an open wound.

Many women become worried when they notice their menstrual blood is a different color or consistency than they've previously experienced, but there's nothing abnormal about having blood that is either red and fresh or brown and clotted. The color and consistency of your period can vary from one cycle to the next, or from day to day within the same period, because blood coagulates. It changes color and consistency when it is outside our blood vessels. Blood is red and runny when it is very fresh, which means it has flowed out of the uterus rapidly and hasn't had time to coagulate. Brown, clotted blood is a bit older. If you have heavy bleeding, it's often fresher because it's easier for the uterus to squeeze it out. If you have very light bleeding, the blood may remain inside the uterus and congeal before flowing out, but the body still gets rid of the coagulated blood, all on its own, in due time. It isn't as if the blood builds up inside you.

A period is neither unhygienic nor dangerous. It consists of blood and mucus and it's up to you how you feel about that. If you want to, there's nothing to stop you from having sex while you're bleeding, but don't forget to use protection. The fact that you're menstruating doesn't mean you're protected against pregnancy or infection by sexually transmitted diseases.

Now that you know what a period is, perhaps you'll understand why we don't usually bleed when we're pregnant—because menstrual blood consists of the mucous membrane that lines the inside of the uterus, which can potentially become the new home of the fertilized egg. When we're pregnant we want to keep this lining so that the fetus won't bleed away. A hormone called progesterone, which you'll soon read more about, helps us keep the mucous membrane in place.

* * *

Hold on a minute, though. You've learned what a period is, but do we actually need it? As you may have noticed, most other female animals don't bleed every single month. A lot of people think female dogs in heat have periods, but that bleeding is something quite different. Female dogs bleed from their vaginas when they're ovulating and able to become pregnant; they don't bleed from the uterus like we do. In fact, periods are a rarity we share with only a couple of human-like apes and some other odd creatures (including a type of bat). In other words, menstruation itself is not a necessity in the animal world in order to have offspring. This is pretty silly—why should we in particular have to waste extra energy making a new uterine lining month after month, again and again, only to see it bleed away to nothing? What's up with that, Darwin?

You've probably heard the terms *evolution* and *natural selection*. Over the history of a species, individuals with random genetic traits that prove advantageous have been particularly successful in transmitting their genes. As a result, these traits dominate in the generations that follow. This is how humans and animals have developed over millennia. Unlike most other mammals, we humans ended up with periods; does that mean that periods themselves constitute an advantage for us? Not according to biologist Deena Emera. Her theory is that periods are not an adaptive advantage, but rather a non-adaptive consequence.[4]

Emera thinks periods are linked to an adaptive advantage that we don't notice in our day-to-day lives: something that we might call spontaneous mucous membrane growth.* The uterine lining grows, as you now know, to provide board and lodging for the fertilized egg. In animals that do not have periods, the mucous membrane only grows when a fertilized egg is present. In other words, the maternal body responds to the cry for help from the fertilized egg by building a uterine lining in which it can live. But

---

* This is a simplification of the term "spontaneous decidualization," which Emera uses in her article. The decidualization process actually involves more than mucous membrane growth.

for humans, the mucous membrane grows spontaneously every month without a fertilized egg being present, and this creates an advantage for us.

When the uterine lining in humans and other menstruating species doesn't receive a fertilized egg, it gets expelled, because there is a cost attached to maintaining extra tissue we don't need. This is why we get periods, which can therefore be described as a consequence of spontaneous growth of the mucous membrane. Animals that don't experience this have no superfluous tissue to get rid of each month, and thus do not have periods. They only produce the lining of the uterus when they need it.

So what is the advantage of spontaneous mucous membrane growth? Emera's theories are based on the idea that the interests of the mother and fetus aren't always aligned—in fact, she suggests that the mother and the fetus have been engaged in an "arms race" over the course of our evolution, in which the fetus develops traits that give it access to more of the mother's resources. The mother, for her part, develops traits that allow her to hold back the resources she needs for her own survival. Against this backdrop, Emera presents two theories about why spontaneous mucous membrane growth is an advantage for humans.

The first is that the growth of the uterine lining protects the mother against an aggressive, invasive fetus, and the fetuses of menstruating species are extra aggressive compared with those that don't have periods. These fetuses have no scruples. They run amok, breaking into their mother's bodies like parasites just to get their hands on energy and nourishment. Since the human has already produced a layer of mucous membrane in advance, this seems to have an extra-protective effect against the invading fetus. You can think of it as the mother having prepared a shield to gain better control over what resources the fetus will have access to and what she'll keep back for herself.

Another theory is that the mother can register the quality of the fetus when the fertilized egg attaches itself to the finished mucous membrane. As you will read in greater detail later on in the book, far from all fertilized eggs end up as babies. Many fetuses are spontaneously aborted at a very early stage because there's something genetically wrong with them. It would be foolish for a mother to waste energy carrying an unviable fetus to term. If she's able to detect this through the lining of the uterus, she can conserve valuable strength by expelling faulty fetuses at an early stage.

The advantage is therefore not the period itself, but the spontaneous mucous membrane growth of which the period is a consequence. Mucous membrane growth is actually only needed for the establishment of a pregnancy; it's not something we require each month. Many people assume that it's important to have bleeding, that it's healthy to have periods, but that's not true. If we cut out the monthly mucous membrane growth, there's no longer any point in having periods. Periods are a consequence and the bleeding is not valuable in itself.

As journalist Lone Frank pointed out in an article about Emera's research, modern human beings are very different from our forebears, who developed monthly menstruation hundreds of thousands of years ago.[5] While modern women have around five hundred cycles over the course of their lives, primitive women would only have had around one hundred. Why? Well, because they spent much of their lives pregnant or breastfeeding in the absence of reliable contraception.

Opting out of periods with the aid of contraception is no more unnatural for us than opting out of having a couple of extra children. Today we have the possibility of choosing whether we want to have children at all, and we can control how many we have. Periods have no intrinsic biological value for modern women.

There are many myths attached to periods; in particular, there's a lot of talk about how periods determine what you can and can't do. But what do periods actually mean to you and your everyday life? Are there some things you should avoid? Is your yoga instructor right, for example, to advise you against doing headstands while your bleeding is at its worst? When we asked a yoga instructor about this, he told us, "It's not good for the blood to run back into your abdominal cavity." In a way, he's right. It's apparently not unusual for small amounts of menstrual blood to run up through the fallopian tubes and out into your abdominal cavity when you have your period. Many stressed-out surgeons have experienced this, finding blood in the abdomen of menstruating women they're operating on without detecting any bleeding wound. It isn't dangerous for menstrual blood to find its way into the belly, though; your body quickly tidies it all up.

Some people also believe that certain activities, such as standing on your head, can cause you to bleed more, but that isn't true either. Periods are the expulsion of the endometrium. You get no more and no less endometrial growth no matter what you do. Over the course of one menstruation, the only thing that bleeds out is the existing endometrial wall. However, the thickness of the wall, and therefore the amount that comes out, may vary from time to time.

Unless particular activities bother you because they cause you pain, you can do exactly what you want when you have your period. You can stand on your head, run a marathon, go swimming, or have sex—it's up to you. Some women even find that physical activity relieves menstrual pains.

But is it really true that we don't bleed more as a result of having sex? When we were writing this chapter at a café in Oslo it occurred to us that we'd both heard stories from our female friends about dramatic and traumatic bleeding that literally caught them with their pants down: there, in the arms of a new male acquaintance, they experienced their heaviest-ever menstrual bleeding. In one case, the woman was woken up, lying in a pool of blood, by a terrified lover who didn't know whether she was dead or alive. *Hello! Helloooo!? Should I call 911?* The incident happened at his house—and the sheets? They were white. In another case, the unexpected bleeding started mid-act, resulting in a scene reminiscent of a slaughterhouse or a 1970s slasher movie. What in heaven's name had happened? We decided to look into this.

It turns out there is no conclusive explanation for what causes these monster bleeds, but there are several theories that may make sense if you know a bit more about how the body works.

The first is what we call "the cramps theory." As we know, muscle contractions in the uterus are what push out period blood; but cramps can be caused by things other than periods. Sometimes uterine cramps aren't bad at all. What we're talking about here is the orgasm, the sexual climax in which the entire sexual apparatus, including the uterus, contracts in fabulous waves. It's possible that an orgasm may kick-start a period that's imminent.

The second theory is the hormone theory. When we have sex, the body releases a hormone called oxytocin, often referred to as the pleasure hormone. Oxytocin plays an important role in various processes in the body. Among other things, it's involved in triggering childbirth in women. Oxytocin stimulates contractions, so it's pretty serious stuff. As if the orgasm alone wasn't enough, oxytocin can also cause the uterus to contract, thereby pushing out blood.

A third possible explanation is that a certain amount of menstrual blood may accumulate inside the vagina and only come out when the "floodgates" open during sex. As you may recall, the vagina contains many folds in which blood can gather. What's more, when you're relaxed, the vagina isn't a hollow tube but a tightly compressed one, whose anterior and posterior walls are squeezed together.

One charming myth that has been making the rounds since the early 1970s is that women's periods synchronize when they live for a long time under the same roof. Our bodies supposedly have some kind of telepathic power that causes us to bond through cramps and chocolate cravings. A Harvard psychologist believed she had proved this after studying the menstrual cycles of women living in the same dorm at an American college.[6] Evolutionary researchers pounced on it, adopting the view that there must be a benefit to women menstruating and ovulating at the same time: men wouldn't be tempted to hop from one woman to another but would form

stable couple relationships instead—a convenient biological explanation for the cultural tradition of monogamy.[7] As many as 80 percent of all women apparently believe in the myth of synchronized
periods.[8]

No matter how cute it sounds, though, more recent research
shows that we've been had. Studies of lesbian couples,[9] Chinese
women living in dorms,[10] and West African women placed in
"menstrual huts" showed no synchronicity.[11] Although we may
seem to be menstruating in sync, this is actually because there's
considerable variation in cycle length from one woman to the next.
If you and your best friend menstruate at the same time, it's most
likely just a matter of chance and not, sadly, a sign that you have a
special bond.

DON'T BLEED ON THE SOFA! ALL ABOUT
SANITARY PADS, TAMPONS, AND MENSTRUAL CUPS

As long as you have access to sanitary products, your monthly
bleeding shouldn't prevent you from doing the stuff you like or
want to do. And the risk of bleeding on your friend's sofa is also
significantly lowered if you stem the flow with something.

The most common hygiene products are disposable sanitary
pads and tampons. Over the past few years, however, the menstrual
cup has been making headway as a favorite for many women. There
are a lot of reasons for this, including economics, the environment,
and comfort. What you choose to use is entirely up to you; it's a
matter of personal taste and your situation.

Women have used different types of sanitary pads ever since we
crept out of the cradle of civilization. One very early (and funny)
description of a pad can be found in a story about the first known
female mathematician. Hypatia, a Greek woman who lived circa
400 AD, is said to have become so sick of a pushy admirer that she
threw her bloody rag at him to put him off.[12] Whether it worked or
not was not reported.

Modern sanitary pads have a self-adhesive strip on the bottom so that you can attach them to your underwear, and they absorb menstrual fluids as they seep out of your vagina. Many different-size pads are available, from tiny thong panty liners to big, soft nighttime pads. The benefit of sanitary pads in comparison with tampons is that you don't risk bacteria growth in your vagina. It's therefore advisable to use pads when the risk of infection is especially high—i.e., in situations where it is easier for bacteria to make their way into the uterus because it is more open, for example just after you've had an intrauterine device inserted, after an abortion, or after childbirth.

A tampon is a small, bullet-shaped object made of absorbent material that you insert into your vagina when you have your period. The advantage of having menstrual protection inside the vagina is that it makes it easier to move about and exercise, and especially to go swimming. Although the word comes from the French tampon, meaning "plug," it doesn't work by keeping the blood inside your vagina. Instead, the tampon collects the blood by absorbing it. Tampons aren't a new invention by any means, but they haven't always come individually wrapped in plastic. Women in ancient Egypt used to insert soft papyrus into their vaginas as menstrual protection.

Today, there are tampons with or without applicators and they come in different sizes. You choose the size according to how much you're bleeding. Keep in mind that there's no point using bigger tampons to avoid having to change them as often—tampons are supposed to be changed frequently; the normal recommendation is to keep a tampon in for three to eight hours. To avoid bacteria growth, it's important to wash your hands thoroughly before changing a tampon.

We've heard tons of tampon stories over the years. One classic involves inserting two tampons at once or "losing" a tampon in your vagina. *Help*, a lot of people think, *now it's going to disappear into my body!* But the idea of a tampon finding its way into your stomach is as much a myth as the idea of a contact lens making its way into your brain through your eye if you're not careful. As you now know, the vagina is an almost completely closed tube. The tiny little passage that runs through the cervix and into the uterus is so narrow that even the smallest tampon could never manage to make its way into the uterus. The cervix is not an open airlock leading into the uterus, and nothing can vanish into your stomach by way of your vagina. Oddly enough, though, things can hide away in the innermost crannies of the vagina and that's why tampons come equipped with a string so that you can pull them out again.

If you're worried that a tampon has gone missing in your vagina, you can try to push it out. Squat and then bear down as if you're going to have a bowel movement. Use your fingers to feel around for it inside. Since the vagina is no more than ten centimeters long, it's usually possible to fish out the tampon yourself. If you can't do it, you need to get yourself to your doctor, ASAP. Tampons that are left in too long are a risk for infection. If you think you're the first person to go to her doctor with this problem, you can set your mind at rest—it's much more common than you may think.

The menstrual cup, a soft silicon beaker that you fold together and insert into your vagina, is a hygiene product that doesn't absorb blood but instead collects it. Once inside, the cup unfolds with its open end toward the cervix. The rim of the cup presses against the vaginal wall, holding it in place. Since the menstrual cup is not a disposable product, hygiene is especially important. It must be emptied, rinsed out, and washed with a mild vaginal rinse at least once every twelve hours. In between each period, it's a good idea to boil the menstrual cup to kill all bacteria.

The primary advantage of the menstrual cup is that you can use it for longer stretches of time than tampons. It's also perfectly fine to exercise and go swimming with a menstrual cup, because it sits inside your vagina. You can use the same menstrual cup for years on end, for up to a decade, which also makes it a cheap and environmentally friendly alternative over time. One menstrual cup can replace thousands of tampons and pads that would otherwise end up in landfills.

As for using tampons, you've almost certainly seen the warnings about proper use. In every single box of tampons, there's a little pamphlet warning against a frightening thing called toxic shock syndrome (TSS).

Toxic shock syndrome is a kind of bacterial infection that attacks the entire body. If you get TSS, you'll notice something is wrong. The symptoms can be high fever, a rash, a sore throat, vomiting, diarrhea, and/or confusion. You'll feel really bad. Incidentally, you should always pay attention to any severe and unexpected symptoms of illness. If you think you have TSS, it's vital to go to the doctor quickly, since the infection will become steadily worse over time and can progress rapidly. In the worst case, the infection can be life-threatening.

Can you really get seriously ill from using tampons? Tampon use is a risk factor for developing TSS because the warm, blood-soaked tampon in the vagina makes a cozy home for bacteria. If you're careless with your hygiene when inserting a tampon and then leave it in for too long, you may be extremely unlucky. This is why it's best not to keep a tampon in for more than eight hours. It takes time for the bacteria to propagate and make their way into the body, so the likelihood of it happening mainly arises if you forget you've got a tampon in your vagina. Proper tampon use is not dangerous.

TSS is a serious disease but also very rare. The proportion of cases of TSS that are caused by tampon use has diminished dramatically since highly absorbent tampons were taken off the market. Today, only around half of the cases of TSS are linked to menstruation. It's also possible to contract TSS from seriously infected wounds and after surgery. In other words, it's quite possible to contract TSS without using tampons, and men can also get it, so perhaps the strong association with tampons is unwarranted.[13]

When it comes to TSS and the menstrual cup, we don't know very much yet because little research has been done on the subject.

The menstrual cup is a relatively new phenomenon. So far, at least one case of TSS linked to the menstrual cup has been reported on a worldwide basis.[14] Although we don't yet know whether the menstrual cup is better or worse than tampons when it comes to TSS, it's always a good idea to pay attention to hygiene.

PMS—PAIN AND MURDER SYNDROME

"What's the matter—got your period?" It's a classic control technique. Sometimes it's a lot easier to write women off as irritable and emotional than to take us seriously. This "period technique" isn't just a sexist way of running women down, it's also wrong, from a strictly physiological point of view. Errors of this kind must be cleared up in the name of popular education. As you may have noticed with your own body, it's not during the days of bleeding that you're most affected psychologically by your menstrual cycle. The problems actually begin *before the bleeding starts*. We're referring, of course, to the well-known if somewhat vaguely defined syndrome, PMS.

PMS, or premenstrual syndrome, may not be fun, but on the whole it's something we can live with. And although it can cause minor problems, PMS isn't a valid reason to write women off in any way whatsoever. Women aren't grouchy, incompetent, or "hormonal" because we have a menstrual cycle. It's possible to behave appallingly regardless of what gender you identify as—we're not disputing that—but blaming someone's bad behavior on their gender is inaccurate and unfair.

PMS is an umbrella term for all the ailments that may arise in the days leading up to your period. They can involve almost anything at all in the way of physical and psychological symptoms: pain, irritability, depression, bloating, mood swings, weeping, anxiety, and acne. The list is a long one. People may also experience a worsening in preexisting illnesses, such as migraine, epilepsy, or asthma. The problems arise in the phase of the menstrual cycle that falls between ovulation and menstruation, what we call the premenstrual or luteal phase. When the period finally arrives, the pressure is relieved and the symptoms evaporate during the first days of bleeding.

There are no specific examinations that can be used to diagnose PMS. The doctor will not be able to tell that you have PMS during a gynecological examination. This makes diagnosis a bit difficult. Your experience of the symptoms is what determines whether or not you have PMS, although minor symptoms in the run-up to your period do not merit the diagnosis. As many as 85 to 95 percent of all women have mild symptoms one or two days before menstruation starts.[15] That is pretty much all of us, and this does not mean that you qualify for a diagnosis or that you need treatment, it just means that you have a female body.

In order to be diagnosed with PMS, then, the symptoms must be of a certain severity. The American College of Obstetrics and Gynecologists says that PMS symptoms must begin at least five days before your period starts and recede within four days after the onset of your period, and your symptoms are not deemed PMS until you experience them for two to three menstrual cycles.[16] They must be so severe that they are a physical or psychological hindrance to your everyday life. Of course, how serious the symptoms are and how much of a hindrance they cause depends on the individual. You can expect some symptoms, but there has to be a limit. Some women are totally incapacitated by their symptoms and that's certainly not the way it should be. As well as being a certain severity, the symptoms must occur during most cycles, i.e., you must have them pretty much every single month. Moreover, the symptoms must stop and start at the times typical for PMS: they must start in the premenstrual phase and stop when your period arrives. Around 20 to 30 percent of all women have symptoms that qualify as mild or moderate PMS.[17]

Women who have the most severe symptoms are generally assigned a diagnosis where the criteria are stricter than for PMS, although many of the same symptoms are still involved. This diagnosis is called PMDD, premenstrual dysphoric disorder; in such cases the symptoms have definitely crossed the line from manageable to unbearable. Irritability, anger, and internal tension are prominent symptoms for these women. This applies to between 3 and 8 percent of all women.[18] There is also a diagnosis known as premenstrual depression. Some women suffer serious signs of depression, such as suicidal thoughts, every single cycle—and this can obviously be dangerous. The three diagnoses overlap somewhat.

Although periods last from puberty to menopause, PMS may not last as long. PMS symptoms can start at any time after your first period, but many women have several PMS-free years in the beginning. Most who suffer from PMS get it by their early twenties, and the symptoms typically continue through the women's entire reproductive lives. Some women experience that the symptoms become more severe later in life, and as a result they do not seek medical help until they are in their thirties or forties.[19] However, when you finally reach menopause, your PMS story is history.[20]

We don't know what causes PMS. Different theories propose everything from higher sensitivity to shifts in the body's hormone levels to neurological or even cultural causes.[21] All women experience hormone swings during their cycle, but why some suffer PMS or PMDD while others are symptom-free is unknown. Perhaps we'll find a cause over time.

Most people don't need medical treatment for PMS and the most important part of the treatment is to avoid medicalizing minor ailments that probably stem from natural hormonal swings in the body. As a rule, PMS is something you can live with and there are alternatives available for people with unbearable problems.

When people suffer severe period issues, treatment is directed at the individual problems, which may vary considerably. If you get depressed or suffer from anxiety, you'll get a different treatment than if you have severe pains. For some people, estrogen-based hormonal contraception can help, allowing them to skip their periods entirely. Other women who suffer primarily from psychological problems may benefit from antidepressants. Those who have pain use painkillers.

Let's go back to the people who resort to sexist control techniques when they speak to women. No matter what you believe, it simply isn't true that women experiencing PMS lose their minds or their capacity to respond rationally in the days before their periods. And if you insist on commenting on where a woman is in her menstrual cycle and using it against her, don't say: "What's the matter—got your period?" but rather, "What's going on? Are you about to have your period in a few days' time?" It doesn't have quite the same ring, but it's important to get your physiology straight if you're going to insult somebody.

THE WHEEL OF ETERNITY—
HORMONES AND THE MENSTRUAL CYCLE

Every month, most fertile women experience an inner, hormone-driven cycle. We're talking about the menstrual cycle. Most of us know a little about it: at some point or another an egg arrives, there's a possibility we may become pregnant if we have sex at the right (or wrong) time, and our period means that we aren't pregnant.

Do we actually need to know any more? We've seen plenty of medical students snap their book shut when they reach the chapter about the menstrual cycle, so why should you bother to read about it? First and foremost, it'll be useful for you; second, it's actually pretty exciting; and third, we promise to make this much easier to grasp than your average textbook author would.

If all of us knew a little bit more about how the minuscule signal substances known as hormones direct us through the menstrual cycle, it would be easier to understand a whole lot of things that all women deal with in their everyday life. We get questions about this all the time: How does hormonal contraception work? What on earth is a fertile window and when does it happen? What controls our menstruation, and what's the mechanism behind various female diseases?

HORMONES—THE SUBSTANCES THAT STEER OUR VESSEL

We ended the section about the internal sex organs with the ovaries and the hormones that are produced there: estrogen and progesterone, the female sex hormones. Now it's time to go into greater detail.

Estrogen has acquired an undeservedly bad reputation lately. All we hear about is the risk of thrombosis, mood swings, the risk of breast cancer, and other scary stuff, but estrogen is actually a fantastic hormone. It's responsible for the things we have traditionally associated with womanliness. Boobs, butt, hips—they're all a result of estrogen. Estrogen is what keeps the vaginal walls moist and thick so that sex feels pleasurable, and it's what makes our uteruses capable of bearing children. It also keeps facial hair and pimples at bay. In fact, transwomen use estrogen treatment to alter the fat distribution on their bodies from the typical male to the typical female distribution. It's pretty incredible what this little hormone can do.

If you've got a feel for language, you can probably work out what progesterone's all about. *Pro* means "for" and *gestation* means "pregnancy." *Progesterone* therefore means "for pregnancy." We need lots of progesterone when our bodies are preparing to receive a fertilized egg, which happens every single month. Progesterone stops the uterus from contracting and pushing out a potentially fertilized egg. In addition, it makes the lining of the uterus an awesome place to live, loading us up with blood and mucus from glands to nourish our future offspring.

Two other hormones are needed to control our menstrual cycle. They come from a pea-sized structure in the brain shaped like a scrotum and called the pituitary gland. (As sex writers, we see sex organs everywhere.)

The brain's two reproductive system hormones are called the follicle-stimulating hormone (FSH) and the luteinizing hormone (LH). Put briefly, the FSH deals with maturation of the egg. The egg actually lies inside a cluster of cells known as a follicle, which accounts for the name "follicle-stimulating hormone." The LH is best known for triggering ovulation. The male brain actually produces precisely the same hormones, but for once the hormones have been named for the function they perform in the female body. Since this is highly unusual in the world of medicine, we think it's extra cool.

So far so good. Now that you've gotten to know the hormones, which are, after all, the stars of this show, it's time to take a look at the cycle itself.

MENSTRUAL CYCLE—TWENTY-EIGHT DAYS AGAIN AND AGAIN AND AGAIN! To understand the menstrual cycle it's useful to draw a circular timeline. Although the length of a cycle can vary from one woman to the next, and even from one period to the next for individual women, we use a model cycle of twenty-eight days for simplicity's sake, since twenty-eight can be neatly divided into four weeks. However, the normal length of a menstrual cycle is between twenty-three and thirty-five days.

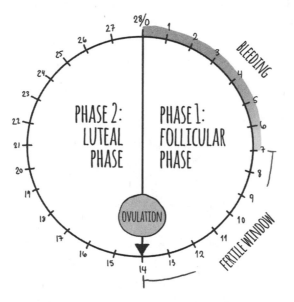

The top of the circle in the drawing marks the beginning of a new cycle and, at the same time, the conclusion of the preceding one. This point is therefore labeled both zero, to symbolize starting over again, and twenty-eight, to indicate that the same point marks the end of the twenty-eighth day, and the conclusion of the previous cycle. The start of one cycle is therefore always simultaneous with the end of another cycle. Your menstrual cycle is a wheel of eternity!

Many people find this difficult to understand. How can the beginning and the end happen at the same time? It's easier to grasp if we compare the menstrual cycle with something that's very familiar to us—this is the exact same thing that happens with a clock when we pass from one day to the next.

At the moment a clock strikes midnight, the time on a digital clock is both 24:00, to mark the last hour of the day that is ending, and at the same time 00:00, to mark a new beginning. The clock moves from one day to the next and on the stroke of midnight, you are in both days at once. There isn't a gap between two days, and the same goes for the menstrual cycle, too.

It's easy to notice the beginning of a new cycle, because that's when you begin to bleed. The bleeding can normally last up to a week, so the first seven days in the cycle.

To keep things straight, the menstrual cycle is often divided into two phases. When you start a new menstrual cycle, you're in what's known as the follicular phase. This is the time when a follicle containing an egg ripens and prepares itself for ovulation. Around day fourteen, marked by the bottom of the circle, comes ovulation, and this marks the transition to phase II, which we call the luteal phase. Half the cycle has now gone by. The next two weeks up until day twenty-eight pass by without any noteworthy events. After twenty-eight days, as you now know, we're back to zero. A new cycle is underway.

Now let's complicate things a bit and imagine that your cycle is thirty days long. In that case, ovulation will happen around day sixteen. Why not on day fifteen, you may be asking? After all thirty divided by two is fifteen. The explanation is that fourteen days pretty much always elapse between ovulation and the first day of the next menstruation. That's the time the body needs to understand whether it has become pregnant or not. If a cycle is longer or shorter than twenty-eight days, this will primarily influence the length of the period *before* ovulation. If you have a very short cycle, you may actually ovulate at the same time as you have your period, although you'll never ovulate on the first day of your period. If you have an irregular cycle, the first day of bleeding is the only day you can know for certain that you won't ovulate.

Now that we have an overview, we can start on the really interesting aspect: the dance of the hormones throughout the cycle. We start at the top of the circle. The period has arrived and we're on the first day of phase one, what's known as the follicular phase. The action isn't isolated to the uterus, because there are also things going on in the ovaries and the brain-scrotum, better known as the pituitary gland. While the uterus is expelling its lining along with all hope of a fertilized egg, the pituitary gland begins to produce FSH. So the brain never gives up; even while the period is underway it's already preparing a new egg and the next shot at pregnancy. As you'll recall, all the eggs in the ovaries lie inside what are known as follicles, which begin to grow once they are stimulated by FSH. The maturation of the follicles is the reason the first phase is called the follicular phase.

So the follicles grow because they receive FSH from the brain, and this in turn causes the follicles to start producing estrogen. As the follicles grow and grow, the quantity of estrogen in the blood begins to increase dramatically. The bigger the follicles, the greater the quantity of estrogen produced. In turn, estrogen influences the uterine lining, causing it to grow. Right after the uterus has finished bleeding, the reconstruction gets underway again. There's no time for a grieving process here. The uterus is a persistent wretch that never passes up an opportunity to receive a fertilized egg, even though it'll be disappointed almost every single month.

While both the follicle and the uterine lining are growing, we approach day fourteen, the day of ovulation and the transition to phase two. The follicle changes shape, becoming a bulging, fluid-filled balloon—a water balloon at bursting point. Now the follicle emits so much estrogen that it sends the levels in the body sky-high—and this is the signal the brain's pituitary gland has been waiting for.

In response to the powerful estrogen signal, the pituitary gland begins to produce LH, the ovulation hormone. We're not talking about small doses here: the quantity of LH suddenly skyrockets. If you've ever tried getting pregnant, it's possible you may be familiar with this dramatic rise in LH. Ovulation tests capture the increase in LH in your urine, so when the ovulation test is positive, you know the rise in LH has started and that ovulation is right around the corner. The immense flow of LH reaches the follicle, which responds by exploding, so that the egg is shot out of its cocoon and out of the ovary. For a little while, the egg floats freely outside the ovary before small tentacles on the fallopian tubes, known as fimbriae, snap it up and send it on a voyage along the fallopian tube toward any sperm cell that may be awaiting it. We are halfway through the menstrual cycle and ovulation is a fact.

Now seems like a good time to take a quick break to comment on a couple of things we didn't learn in high school biology class. It's about the egg cell. You probably remember the heroic battle or race between the tough-guy sperm cells, which swim frantically to be the first to fertilize the waiting, passive egg. Point one: the egg doesn't stand still. The egg doesn't hang around nervously in the bar waiting for the sperm cell. The egg is a diva and, like most divas, she tends to turn up at the party fashionably late. As we'll discuss more in the section on pregnancy, the best time to have sex in order to become pregnant is in the days *before* ovulation. The egg isn't passive at all. It's at least as active as the sperm cell. It isn't the sperm cells that swim toward the egg but rather the egg that comes bobbing down toward the waiting sperm cells. They've often been waiting for her for days . . .

Point two: an equally heroic battle is waged between the egg cells as between the sperm cells, but for some reason or another, we don't talk about that in school. Follicle-stimulating hormones (FSH) don't just affect one egg follicle each month. As you now know, up to a thousand follicles begin to grow and mature every single month, but only one of the very largest ones will have the pleasure of exploding and releasing its egg. The other eggs wither away and die without ever having the chance to meet a sperm cell. Now perhaps you think a thousand follicles competing isn't as tough as what the sperm cell is exposed to—after all, they have to race against millions! Remember, though, that men produce many millions of sperm cells every single day, whereas we women are born with all the eggs we'll ever have. And they run out.

Why is it so natural to present egg cells (from women) as passive and sperm cells (from men) as active when this absolutely doesn't correspond to reality? Just wondering . . .

But back to the menstrual cycle. We're in phase two, i.e., days fifteen to twenty-eight on the timeline, or the luteal phase. The egg has just been released and the uterine lining has grown nice and thick thanks to all the estrogen from the follicles. In phase two, progesterone is the star hormone, whereas in phase one, it was estrogen that caused the uterine lining to grow. Progesterone is produced from the remains of the punctured follicle in which the egg lived before it was released. The remains of the follicle change shape and color, becoming a little cluster known as the corpus luteum, which is Latin for yellow body, so called because of its yellow color. Sometimes things are that simple.

As we said earlier, *progesterone* means "for pregnancy," so now the body takes the final steps to prepare itself to receive the fused egg and sperm cells. The progesterone prevents the uterus from contracting and expelling the endometrium, at the same time ensuring that the uterine lining is an extra-comfy place to live.

Meanwhile, the pituitary gland is prevented from producing FSH or LH, i.e., the hormones that make new eggs develop and grow. After all, we don't need to mature new eggs when we hopefully have a fertilized egg on the way! Progesterone from the corpus luteum is what blocks the pituitary gland in this way.

Unfortunately (for the corpus luteum), phase two of the menstrual cycle almost always ends in a tragic tale of suicide, as we will now see. The progesterone from the corpus luteum stops the pituitary gland from producing any FSH and LH, but the problem is that the corpus luteum needs both of these hormones to survive. In other words, the corpus luteum prevents production of its own life preserver and will only be rescued if fertilization takes place. Most often, therefore, the corpus luteum falls victim to its own altruistic struggle to keep the potentially fertilized egg alive. Without fertilization, the corpus luteum fades away and dies, and the progesterone vanishes along with it, too.

With the corpus luteum out of the way, there's no longer any progesterone preventing the pituitary gland from doing what it's best at: producing hormones. The level of FSH and LH in the blood rises again, and the follicles in the ovaries get to work once more, ready for a new opportunity to mature, explode, and let their eggs fuse with one chosen sperm cell. Without progesterone from the corpus luteum there's nothing to retain the thick endometrium or prevent the uterus from contracting. We know the outcome: the period. The first day of bleeding. We're back at the top of the circle. The cycle is over, but a new one has already started.

WHEN CAN YOU ACTUALLY GET PREGNANT?

It's a given that sex must happen in order for women to get pregnant naturally, but beyond that, there seems to be a great deal of uncertainty. In one episode of the reality TV show *Paradise Hotel* (a show that aired in the United States in 2003 and never really took off, but has been wildly popular in Norway since our version premiered in 2009), a lively discussion started over the breakfast table after two of the participants had had unprotected sex: "What if she gets pregnant?" Some stubbornly insisted that everything would be fine because the woman in question had just had her period, while others claimed that women were most fertile right after menstruation. The confusion was total and the solution turned out to be emergency contraception funded by the TV network. This pregnancy business isn't simple.

Pregnancy is a watershed in women's lives. We can go from being terrified of it and expending a considerable amount of brainpower on how best to avoid it to wishing for it so much that it can't happen quickly enough. It's the worst and the best that can happen to us, depending on where we are in life and who we are with. It may therefore seem remarkable to write a section about pregnancy that will serve both groups, but it's actually very simple. Knowledge about how we become pregnant is the best medicine whether you want to prevent pregnancy or wish to become pregnant. So what does it take?

Let's start off by stating the obvious. You can't get pregnant from anal sex, oral sex, or from sitting on a toilet seat with sperm on it (yuck). You must have vaginal sex, i.e., sex with your vagina. After that, it gets a bit more complicated.

When a man has an orgasm during vaginal sex, many millions of sperm cells are squirted up into the woman's vagina. Most of them die after a short time; the majority by running out of the vagina after sex or by swimming off into some dark corner of the vagina. Very few sperm cells manage to find the cervical opening, and even then it's all a matter of timing.

Most of the time, the cervical opening is, in fact, closed by a thick, gelatinous mucus plug that the body produces in response to naturally high levels of the hormone progesterone. Only in the time around ovulation does the mucus plug dissolve, opening the passageway into the uterine cavity. In the days before ovulation, you may actually notice this since your discharge changes, containing elastic threads of mucus! This mucus, which is similar to egg whites, can be stretched to incredible lengths between your fingers, if you're curious about trying.

When ovulation approaches, the progesterone level diminishes and the body produces more of the estrogen hormone. Estrogen causes the cervical opening to produce a runny, watery fluid instead of gelatinous slime, and this makes it possible for the sperm cells to swim up into the uterine cavity. Again, you can observe this from your discharge, which becomes more runny and milky. That is when you are ovulating and at your most fertile.

Let's say you have unprotected sex in that window around ovulation when your cervix is open. A little gang of a couple of hundred sperm cells have managed to find their way into your uterus. They will now spend between two and seven hours moving through the uterus and up into one of the fallopian tubes. They're helped along by small, rhythmic movements in the uterus and fallopian tubes, which create waves the sperm can surf along on. Their choice of direction is vital, because the eggs almost always come from one ovary at a time. Once inside the fallopian tube, the sperm cells take a rest and wait for the egg—because, as you now know, the egg is clearly the diva of the party, and she keeps the sperm cells waiting. Sperm cells normally survive in the uterus or fallopian tubes for about forty-eight hours, although living sperm cells have actually been found as many as five to seven days after sexual intercourse. Who knew sperm were so hardy and patient?

After ovulation, the egg will bob down along the fallopian tube toward the waiting sperm. Fertilization occurs when one sperm cell fuses with one egg in the fallopian tube and together they create the precursor of a fetus, known as a zygote. Now and then two eggs will be released during ovulation and then you may get two-egg twins (known as "fraternal twins"). This happens more often as women age, and it is also hereditary, so that some families will have several sets of twins. In rare cases, a set of one-egg twins (considered "identical twins") may be born. This happens when the zygote splits into two separate pieces immediately after being fertilized by a sperm cell.

One day after fertilization, the fertilized egg is still floating around in one of the fallopian tubes, but now the cells have begun to divide. Even so, this is no guarantee that you will become pregnant. In order for the pregnancy to be successful, the growing cluster of cells must find its way down into the uterus and attach itself to the mucous membrane on the wall of the uterus at the right time. In addition, the body must receive a signal from the uterus indicating that the cluster of cells is in place via a hormone called hCG—the same hormone that pregnancy tests measure in the urine. This is the hormone that ensures that the corpus luteum we spoke about in the menstrual cycle section (pages 65–7) survives and continues to produce progesterone. If this doesn't happen, the fertilized egg will be flushed out with the next menstruation without you noticing a thing.

It takes between seven and ten days after fertilization for the cluster of cells to attach itself to the lining of the uterus. Only then are you actually pregnant. The next forty weeks or so are such an extensive journey that we have opted to skip them. After all, there are plenty of pregnancy books available for you to read.

Back to our *Paradise Hotel* couple. Is the woman likely to have become pregnant if she's just had her period? In a study of couples who were trying for a baby, only those who'd had sex during a six-day window around ovulation achieved pregnancy, i.e., five days before ovulation plus the day of ovulation itself.[22] Those who had sex the day before ovulation or the day on which it occurred had a 30 percent chance of becoming pregnant. Five days before ovulation, 10 percent became pregnant.

So a significant number became pregnant even though they had sex long before ovulation. As mentioned, sperm cells can survive in a woman's body for up to a week before dying, so, in theory, you're fertile for a period ranging from seven days before ovulation until one day afterward, i.e., a total of eight days. In other words, we have an eight-day fertile window. Most of us aren't aware of our ovulation, so the key to knowing whether the *Paradise* participant was in the risk zone would have been to map her cycle to see how long it was.

As we described in the section on the menstrual cycle, ovulation most often occurs fourteen days before the next menstruation. If you have a totally stable cycle of twenty-eight days, ovulation will always occur in the middle of the cycle, on the fourteenth day, or two weeks after your last period started. Given the eight-day window, this means it's possible for you to become pregnant between days eight and fifteen of your cycle.

Let's say that the *Paradise* participant has a stable twenty-eight-day cycle and a period that lasts seven days, i.e., days one to seven in the cycle. That'll mean she has only one, just one single day after her period before her chance of becoming pregnant arises. Five days after she's had her period, there's a considerable chance of her becoming pregnant.

In such a cycle, it definitely won't be safe to have unprotected sex when she's just had her period. In the week before she's expecting her next period, days twenty-one to twenty-eight, however, it will be safe. We can thank emergency contraception or sheer luck for the fact that there was no *Paradise* baby.

It may sound as if it should be pretty simple to figure out what your safe periods are if you can only get pregnant eight days in every cycle. The problem is that very few women have entirely stable cycles. You've probably noticed this yourself, too. Since you never know in advance whether you'll ovulate sooner or later than normal this month, you have to operate with a wider window. If ovulation shifts either backward or forward by just two days, this will lengthen the unsafe period to twelve days. Many women have greater variation than this. If, in addition, you're the kind of person who doesn't like having sex during her period, you're left with just a few days when you can have sex without using contraception and still be confident that you won't get pregnant. In other words, it's sensible to always use contraception.

PART 3: SEX

If there's one thing we humans have had in common since the dawn of time, it's sex. Most of us have had or will have sex, both with ourselves and with other people. Without sex, there would be no more humans on Earth, and we think humans would have had much more boring lives. Sex is one of the most natural things we can do. Even the way we have sex—whether homosexual or heterosexual—isn't so different from other animals.

The difference is that the human race is the only species that's ashamed of having sex. We hide away when we do it—or at least that's the norm. This secrecy means sex has always been clouded in uncertainty. We don't know what everybody else is doing, we don't know if our desires are normal, and we can never be quite certain that we measure up. Paradoxically enough, even though we usually do it as a twosome, sex is a pretty lonesome business. This is especially true when you're at the very beginning of your sex life, in puberty.

A great deal is written about sex these days, and many young people spend hours watching porn. Sex videos are shared on social media and teens send snaps of hard penises and erect nipples to people they're involved with. Some might claim we're living in the most openly sexualized society ever.

As such, a remarkable duality now exists. We have unique access to inspiration and insight about our desires and bodies. Knowledge is just a mouse click away. At the same time, this openness doesn't seem to have made us any more confident; quite the opposite.

The problem is that what we are initiated with is a glossy version. Ideals about sex have been raised, but at the same time the uncertainty lives on inside us. We still want to shy away when we're turned on, but our environment tells us that everything should be shared. The contrasts can feel overwhelming. The result, we believe, is that a lot of women feel as if their libidos are too low and they have too little exciting sex and too few orgasms.

There's a need for a new understanding of reality. Here we want to talk about what we understand a normal sex life to be. And, of course, when we use the word *normal*, we don't mean to say anything that falls outside this is wrong or something to be ashamed of; it's just not what most people do. Sexuality comes in a thousand forms and only you know what's right for you. We hope to add nuance to the way we think about sex and to offer some tips about how to find your way to a satisfying and stress-free sex life.

FIRST-TIME SEX

Few experiences in life are so veiled in legend as "doing it," having sex, for the first time. Your expectations about performance—your own and your partner's—can be sky-high and it's difficult to imagine what lies ahead.

As a result, some people are disappointed in themselves or their partner after their first sexual experience. Didn't you have an orgasm? Was it difficult to get into the positions you'd read about? Did your boyfriend's penis go soft after ten seconds? Didn't she touch your clitoris?

Courage! Sex is like most other things in life. You don't get good at it without practice, and nor does your partner. It's important to bear in mind that the first time won't be perfect, but if you lower your expectations a bit, it can still be a positive experience. There's got to be a first time, after all. We've collected a bit of information that may help make that first time as good as possible.

In the film *Just Bea* (2004), we follow a group of friends in the first year of high school in Oslo. Bea is the only one who hasn't done it yet. One of the rituals in her group of girlfriends is that you get a piece of marzipan cake from the local bakery once you've lost your virginity. Bea is now sixteen years and nine months old, and she feels as if everything depends on whether or not she can get laid. The slice of marzipan cake in the bakery window is calling out to her.

Bea isn't the only one out there who thinks "everyone else has done it," that there's some rush to get it out of the way. When these kinds of thoughts pop up, it's handy to have a few facts on the table.

The average age for both Norwegian and American women to have sex for the first time is around seventeen,[1] but that's just an average, not a prescription. Some people start earlier, some later. In fact, only 20 percent of all young people start having sex before they're sixteen, and a study by the Guttmacher Institute found that the number of teenagers who have sex for the first time at age fifteen and younger has decreased in recent years.[2] So four out of five young people haven't had sex when they start their first year of high school. In other words, there's no need for Bea to be in a hurry for that slice of cake.

Although it may be good to have an average age to relate to, it's important to remember that your first time is about you and your partner. You should start having sex when you're *both* ready for it. You're ready when you feel desire (desire is in your head), and when you are turned on (this is in your body). Now and then, your head and body might not be on quite the same page, and in that case it may be a good idea to wait a while. When we get turned on and who makes us feel that way varies from person to person. Some people feel ready when they're in high school, others when they're in college, and others wait until they're in their twenties or even older.

Most people have sex for the first time with a partner of their own age. Some people do it with their girl- or boyfriend, others with a one-night stand, others with a buddy, male or female. For some people it happens in a bedroom, for others, in the back seat of a car. None of these things are wrong, as long as everybody involved actually wants to play the game.

Just remember that the Cardamom Law applies:* you and your partner may be hot to have sex RIGHT NOW, but it may be best to wait to have sex in a place and at a time that isn't going to bother other people. For example, it isn't fun to sit next to a couple having sex on a plane. Ellen can vouch for this, having experienced it on a flight to New York. The fact that these lovebirds pretended to speak neither English nor Norwegian when they were clearly from Kristiansand (a town in southern Norway) only made the situation worse. Have respect for each other *and* those around you.

A lot has been said and written about what constitutes "losing" one's virginity. Is it possible to engage in some sexual activities and still be a virgin? Are you a virgin if you've had anal but not vaginal sex? What about oral sex or fingering? What counts as *real* sex? We don't have the answer to that, but we believe there's far too much focus on labeling things. There's no wrong or right consensual sex; and there's no sex that is more or less "real." You're the one who decides the terms of your sex life. First-time sex can actually be so many things, since sex includes oral sex, fingering, vaginal, and anal sex. You can have fantastic sex without having traditional vaginal intercourse. After all, it's totally absurd to claim a lesbian is a virgin until she's had vaginal sex with a man.

Most young people today know a fair amount about what sex involves. This isn't only due to sex education, because most of them have actually seen sex in the form of pornography.[3] Despite (or perhaps because of?) this, a lot of young people are worried about whether they're "good enough" at sex before they do it the first time.

The first time you have sex, you can expect it to involve a lot of flailing. No matter what you do, it's not going to be like it is in a porno. Like other films, some porn uses effects so that things look

---

* The Cardamom Law, from Thorbjørn Egner's Norwegian children's book *When the Robbers Came to Cardamom Town* translates roughly as: Don't bother other people, be both good and kind, other than that feel free to do whatever comes to mind.

different than they do in reality, and there's a lot of make-believe going on. So it isn't possible to do all the things you see in porn movies in real life, even though porn is inspired by and based on something that's real. It's a bit like the Hobbit films: there may be mountains in real life, but that doesn't mean there are dragons living in them. And even if there were, they wouldn't have Benedict Cumberbatch's voice.

It's also important to remember that porn actors should be viewed as extreme athletes. They've done it all before, so to speak. Lindsey Vonn makes downhill skiing look easy, but you'd probably have broken your neck if you tried to imitate her the first time you put on a pair of skis.

Don't expect to be able to perform like Stoya, the famous porn actor. You won't be able to achieve advanced Kama Sutra positions on your first attempt. You'll probably never manage them at all, and that's fine: you don't need to in order to have good sex. It will be pretty clumsy the first time, but that's the way it's supposed to be. That's part of the charm. You'll almost certainly feel as if you have one arm too many or two legs too few, but it'll get easier with practice.

It isn't just important to lower your expectations about your own performance. Remember to cut your partner some slack, too. He or she won't know what you like the first time you have sex together and will probably be at least as nervous as you are. In any event, it may be good to talk about it afterward, even have a debriefing. What worked? Will there be a next time? If so, what should you do differently?

HOW AM I SUPPOSED TO GET ANYTHING IN THERE?

Sex is, indeed, so many things and an exaggerated focus on vaginal intercourse excludes too many people. After all, sex doesn't have to be between a woman and a man, although it may often seem that way in our heteronormative society. In Norway, around one in ten women have had sexual experience with somebody of their own gender.[4] In the United States, where adolescent females are more likely than their male peers to report a same-gender sexual partner, a review of Youth Risk Behavior Surveillance data gathered from eight US sites from 2001 to 2009 concluded that students who identified as lesbian or gay were more likely (median 67 percent) than students who identified as heterosexual (median 44 percent) to ever have engaged in sexual intercourse.[5] With that in mind, we'll give a little extra space here to first-time vaginal sex. Not because it's the only way to have sex, but because it's what we get the most questions about.

An incredible number of girls ask themselves the following questions before they have vaginal sex: Will I bleed? Will it hurt? A lot of women are afraid their vaginas will be too tight. How am I supposed to fit anything in there? I can't even get a tampon in!

The idea of getting something as big as a penis into a vagina may seem dramatic, but there's actually plenty of room. Your vagina is incredibly flexible and can expand in all directions when you're turned on. A lot of people think women who haven't had sex have tighter vaginas than those who have. You've probably heard that your vagina gets saggier and saggier the more you have sex. That's not true.

The vagina is a powerful muscular tube and you yourself can actually regulate how tight it will be. This regulator works regardless of how many penises or dildos you've had in your vagina. If you really relax, it'll be easier for a penis to slip in, but if you clench, it may be difficult to get *anything* in there. Even if you've had sex a lot of times, you can still tighten your vagina and make it narrower. If you use your vaginal muscles actively during sex, you can regulate the friction between the vagina and the penis. Just experiment!

A lot of girls are nervous before having vaginal sex for the first time and that's hardly surprising, given all the pressure of expectation. It's perfectly fine to be a little nervous, but if you're too nervous, it can make the experience an unpleasant one. When you're nervous, it's easy to unconsciously tighten the muscles in your vagina, making it difficult to get anything in there. That can make it hurt a bit.

When women get turned on, their genitals often react by producing more moisture. This slick fluid serves as the body's natural lubrication.* If you're very stressed, it's difficult to get turned on and wet. This can happen even if you've actually decided that you want to have sex. In a way, nervousness can prevent your body from going along with what you want.

If you're dry or you're involuntarily tightening your vagina, it's easy to get small tears in the vaginal wall that may bleed slightly. It's not dangerous, but it can be unpleasant and sting. The key is to take it easy the first time. Spend time on kissing and foreplay, so that it's easier for your muscles to relax. Give yourself time to be really turned on, and that way you'll also produce more moisture.

Some girls don't get wet regardless, even if they relax, spend time on foreplay, and want to have sex. On the other hand, some women get wet when they actually don't feel aroused. There isn't always a link between the brain and the genitals. The great thing is that there are alternatives to the vagina's natural moisture. It's equally good to use spit, or lubricant from the supermarket or drugstore. Lubricant may improve a lot of people's experience and it might be a good idea to have some around the first time, when you don't know exactly how your body is going to react.

And then there's the hymen, unfortunately also known as the virginal membrane. As discussed, it's the narrowest part of the vagina, but we might as well repeat some of the particulars. Your hymen won't necessarily bleed the first time you have sex. It's roughly as likely that you won't bleed as that you will. And nobody will be able to tell from looking at your genitals afterward whether you've had sex or not. There's no vaginal membrane to rupture, just a flexible ring of tissue. Don't waste energy worrying about your hymen. Spend time worrying about serious things instead, like the environmental crisis, the refugee situation, and the lack of quality sex education in schools. Your hymen isn't worth losing sleep over.

---

*   This doesn't apply to all women. It's quite possible to be turned on without getting wet and vice versa. You can be wet without feeling any desire whatsoever. You can read more about that in the section on desire (pages 95–106).

TIPS AND TRICKS

You now know a lot about what happens in the vagina when you have sex, but how are you supposed to go about doing it from a practical point of view? We have two suggestions for how you can have vaginal sex for the first time, from a strictly technical standpoint, but you may well opt for a third alternative. It's your vagina, after all. The alternatives are different, but equally good.

The first is super traditional, but definitely worth considering. The missionary position isn't often used in porn because you see so little of the sex organs (and what would porn be without exposed sex organs?), but in the real world, missionary is a winner when you're having sex for the first time. The missionary position involves you (the female) lying on your back while the guy lies between your legs, so that your chests and stomachs are facing each other. The penis goes into your vagina when the guy moves back and forth on top of you. It's not an active position from your point of view, but there are several reasons why this is a good place to start. You have full access to and oversight of each other's bodies; you can kiss as you go along; and, last but not least, it's possible for you to observe each other's reactions, so you always know if the other person's having a good time (or not). This is especially important the first time, when both of you are nervous. If there's too much eye contact, you can just shut your eyes.

Some find it scarier to give up control than to simply take charge. A lot of people are scared shitless of being driven along the highway by other people and feel the need to be back-seat drivers. Are you like that? If so, it's much better for you to take control yourself. We'll put you on top. A good starting point is for the guy to lie on his back and you to lie on top of him. It's a bit like a reverse missionary position. Place your knees on either side of his hips and sit on his penis. If you like, you can give yourself extra support by resting your lower arms or hands on the bed. You absolutely don't have to sit as if you were on a horse, even though people often talk about this position as the woman "riding" the man, or cowgirl position. If you feel too exposed sitting upright, you can lean forward. If you like it that way, you can ride on. Now you're the one who's going to do most of the moving. You yourself can control how deep the penis slides into your vagina and how quickly things will go. That's the advantage of sitting on top! As with the missionary position, you have a good view of each other's faces when you're on top. Yes, it can be a bit scary, but it's easier to communicate if something's good or bad.

Not all sex ends in orgasm, although that may be the impression you get from porn or Hollywood films. This applies to both males and females. Orgasm is something that comes with practice and not something you should expect of yourself or your partner the first time you have sex. In order to have an orgasm, it's important to know your own body well and to feel safe. For those reasons, some women seem to find it easier to have an orgasm with a person they're in a steady relationship with. Another important way to get to know your own body is to masturbate. For a lot of people, it takes several years to manage to have an orgasm with their sex partners: it's often easier to come when you do it all by yourself, but practice makes perfect! We'll come back to that (page 106).

Communication with your partner is very important. By all means say what you want, but don't expect him or her to be able to figure out your orgasm for you. It's perfectly fine and normal to take things into your own hands. Having sex with a partner doesn't mean you can't devote attention to yourself at the same time. After all, you can show your partner what you're doing and then your partner can show you what he or she likes.

Sex is fun, but like other fun things, there's a risk attached. In the same way that seat belts and bicycle helmets reduce the risk of serious injury, contraception reduces the risk of sexually transmitted diseases and pregnancy.

Contraception is definitely a shared responsibility. If it takes two to have sex, it takes two to decide on and commit to contraception. It's never sensible to assume that your partner will come prepared. Our advice to you is to always take matters into your own hands. That's also our advice to any young men who might be reading this.

If your partner is prepared, too, that's a good sign. It may mean this is a person with a good head on their shoulders.

Contraception requires planning, so find out how to use it well before having sex for the first time. Seek guidance from a doctor or nurse and take a look at our chapter on contraception (page 119). Everything you need to know is in there. We recommend combining condoms with a contraceptive method that protects well against pregnancy. For now, the contraceptive alternatives offered are almost exclusively for women. The condom is the only form of contraception that offers protection against sexually transmitted disease. By all means use a condom on its own, but make sure it doesn't get damaged when you're in the middle of the act (follow our condom course later on, pages 132–3). It may also be a good idea to have a morning-after pill on hand or know where you can get one in case something goes wrong. You'll learn more about that soon (pages 138–44).

If you want to have sex and you have the contraception situation under control, go right ahead. You're the only person who knows whether you're ready or not. Nonetheless, our most important advice is to take the first time for what it is: *the first time*. There'll be plenty of others; you'll become more skillful and it will get better.

ANAL SEX

We closed the section called "The Other Hole" with a real cliffhanger: The area around and right inside your anus is full of nerve endings just waiting to be stimulated. Some people find that it expands the dimensions of their sex life if they invite their butt to the party.

Great—we have lots of anal nerve endings, but how are we supposed to go about stimulating them? Perhaps you think it sounds a bit overoptimistic to "invite your butt to the party." Lots of people think anal sex sounds scary and kind of dirty; in the same category as whips and blindfolds. "What? Are we supposed to have sex with the same hole we poop out of?"

Anal sex is undoubtedly "Sex 201": advanced sex. It's not something you have to do if aren't into it. Nonetheless, it's becoming steadily more common among heterosexual couples. In 2013, a study found that nearly one in five of all young Brits aged sixteen to twenty-four had had anal sex in the previous year.[6] There's no reason to think young people elsewhere are any different.

So people have anal sex, but they often have it for the wrong reasons. Unfortunately, it's been observed that anal sex is all too often an activity that girls are pressured into having and that they experience as unpleasant or painful.[7] There's a widespread perception that anal sex is something girls must "learn to enjoy." That's not the way it should be. Anal sex should be voluntary and it should be good. If you're not interested, don't pursue it. Set your own boundaries.

If you are curious, however, read on. Many women like anal sex, which can be so many things. The term includes all types of stimulation of the anus. It may entail penetrative sex with a penis or a dildo, and it may involve fingering or oral sex—licking on and around the anus, which is also known as *rimming*. The fact that you don't relish the thought of a penis in your butt doesn't mean you can't find other ways to get pleasure from your anus.

The advice in this section deals with penetrative anal sex, i.e., with fingers, penis, or other objects. Since having butt sex is a bit different from having vaginal sex, there are a few things you need to know before you get started.

As you may remember from earlier, the anus has two strong, adjoining sphincters: one that works automatically without you doing anything at all, and another one that's a voluntary muscle. This is practical because it means we aren't constantly having to dash to the bathroom for a number two. The sphincter keeps the anus tight, making it as wrinkled as a pleated skirt and concealing the actual size of the ring.

A lot of people think the anal canal and rectum are very narrow and much tighter than the vagina. This may be one of the reasons for its apparently magical power of attraction for men, but it's only a partial truth. The rectum is actually like a balloon: just tied shut at one end with a knot. The sphincters are at the very end and press the end of the gut together with immense force. This means that it is extremely narrow at the very end, but once you get past the sphincters there's plenty of room. The vagina, on the other hand, is a tube full of muscles all the way from the vaginal opening up to the cervix. So the vagina can be narrow all the way up, whereas the rectum is mostly narrow right at the end. What's more, it isn't as if the sphincters are narrow all the time. After you've been going at it for a little while, they relax so that the rectum isn't especially narrow at any point.

The balloon knot means that anal sex involves some very particular challenges. When you're going to have vaginal sex, we talk about "relaxing" so the pelvic muscles won't contract and make it difficult to have sex. The sphincters in the anus don't work in the same way. As you know, your butt is still closed when you are totally relaxed. It remains closed even when you're sleeping or in deep meditation. This is the involuntary ring muscle at work. You can't actively make the opening larger by relaxing. What you can do is prevent the voluntary sphincter from contracting as well. You have no control over the involuntary sphincter but, as we've said, it will gradually become looser with stimulation.

The most important advice, therefore, is to take it easy in the beginning. Don't launch yourself at a hard penis or a massive dildo if you've never had anything up your back passage before. It takes time for the sphincters to relax. First you have to get the voluntary muscles that you can control to relax, and after that the involuntary sphincter has to take the hint. Start out by inserting smaller things, fingers or smaller sex toys, and get used to the feeling. Most people need to warm up for a considerable amount of time before they're ready for the, ahem, big one.

If you take it too fast, the anus is prone to small tears that can be horribly painful in the days following the act. Anybody who's ever aimed for the vagina but ended up with the full length of their partner in the wrong hole instead knows all about that. It hurts. If you're going to have anal sex, you must be ready for it. This also means that your partner must be prepared to be incredibly patient. Just going for it won't work here.

Once you're underway, things get easier. Your anus becomes more and more slack—and that brings us to something a lot of people find scary. The balloon knot doesn't close up once you're finished. "Oh no! Is my ring going to be saggy forever?" Far from it—relax. The muscles do slowly tighten again, it just takes a bit of time.

It's true that it is possible to permanently injure the sphincters, in the same way that it's possible to injure any part of your body. But you'd have to give them a real pummeling. Remember that the anus is designed to expel larger things than your average penis. Start off calmly, proceed carefully, and stop if anything feels wrong: that way everything will be fine.

Another important aspect of anal sex is moisture. While the vagina usually becomes wet of its own accord when you're aroused, you have to use lubricant or some equivalent type of artificial moisture to have anal sex. Without lubricant, it'll be difficult to get anything in and if it's too dry, there'll be a lot of friction. Friction increases the risk of tears and light bleeding.

It's true that a little bit of moisture is produced by the glands in the rectum, but that happens regardless of whether or not you're turned on. The inside of your gut has a mucous membrane, just like the inside of your vagina and mouth. The hallmark of mucous membranes is that they produce moisture: spit in the mouth and vaginal secretions in the vagina. When the mucous membrane in the rectum is irritated by, say, a penis, it produces mucus to protect itself against damage. So sex in itself will trigger the production of some moisture, but it isn't enough. You need lubricant as well.

Now on to the big question: feces, poop, number two. We've all heard urban legends about women who've accidentally defecated on their partners during anal sex. It's hardly a tempting prospect for most of us, but there's no getting away from the fact that there is feces in the rectum. Even if you don't feel as if you need to defecate, feces accumulate in the bowel until it is full. The rectum is a storage place for poop before it escapes into the outside world. This means feces can end up on a penis, sex toy, or finger and if you haven't thought about it in advance, it may come as a shock. If it does happen, there's nothing wrong with it and no reason for you to feel embarrassed. If you're going to have anal sex, that's part of the game.

It is, however, possible to reduce the risk of the appearance of feces. Some people choose to use enemas to flush out their rectum, but doctors don't recommend this because they can disturb normal gut flora and make you more susceptible to sexually transmitted infections. Take care to empty your bowels and wash up before you get going.

You cannot, of course, become pregnant from having butt sex, but you absolutely can get sexually transmitted diseases from doing it. Some people forget this, or believe they're less likely to be infected in the anus. In fact, it's quite the opposite. Many sexually transmitted diseases (not just HIV) are more easily transmitted through anal sex, partly because anal sex is more likely to result in tears or bleeding than other types of sex. If you have sex with new partners, it's important to use a condom until you and your partner have been tested. This applies regardless of what kind of sex you have.

As you know, it's fine to have vaginal sex without a condom after you and your partner have been tested for sexually transmitted infections (STIs), but your butt contains bowel bacteria, so hygiene is important! You don't want to get bowel bacteria into your vagina or your urethra where they don't belong, because that can lead to infections. So be careful when you're switching straight from anal to vaginal sex, with either finger or penis. It's a good idea to use a condom during anal sex and take it off and put on a fresh one if you want to continue with vaginal sex. Remember to clean the sex toys you use anally as well.

Incidentally, there are toys designed especially for anal use. They often have a plug at one end to prevent them from disappearing right up into your rectum. Nothing can disappear in the vagina, because it is no more than seven to ten centimeters long and is closed at the top. However, the bowel is endless, practically speaking. It's pretty awful to have to go to the ER to remove objects that have gotten stuck, but it does happen. Doctors get a tremendous amount of enjoyment out of exchanging stories about all the strange things they've had to fish out of people's backsides: chunky candles, toy cars, iPods, or bottles. Doctors are allowed their fun, too.

This was a primer for those of you who want to try anal sex. Done properly, it can be wonderful for women and men alike, but for that to happen, women must stop doing it for men's sake. Anal sex, like all other sex, should only happen because you both want to do it.

A TOTALLY NORMAL SEX LIFE

When *Girls* (2012–17) first took our TV screens by storm, many people described it as revolutionary to finally see normal women having normal sex—whatever that is. Instead of multiple orgasms and steamy sex on the kitchen counter, we got to see clumsiness, awkward pauses, and failed attempts to show up at boyfriends' houses wearing sexy underwear. It's striking how hard the girls in the series try to live up to the sexual ideals of popular culture, with wildly varying degrees of success. Dirty talk and spanking seemed sexy in the latest *Elle* article, but when Adam and Hannah try it in real life, it turns into the very best kind of cringe TV. *Girls* is the clash between the ideal and the reality.

Girls was a reaction to the fact that sex has become public property. People talk loud and long over bottles of red wine about the most intimate details of their friends' sex lives. Women have taken ownership of sex. It's cool to be into having sex, cool to know what you want. And that's great, for those who achieve it.

Unfortunately, expectations about how your sex life ought to be come along as part of the baggage. Our sex lives have become yet another arena where we are supposed to perform. Only in a tête-à-tête with a good female friend do the more sensitive and private questions come out: Is it normal to only have sex every other week? Do you give your boyfriend a blow job every time you have sex? Am I abnormal if I can only come by touching myself during sex?

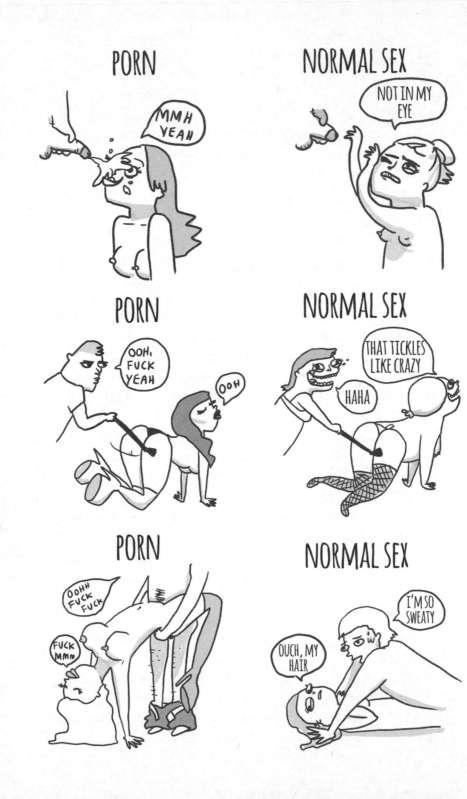

Because, what actually constitutes a normal sex life? We went on a quest to discover standard sex.

When people are assessing their sex lives, the *amount* of sex is generally the easiest aspect to compare with others. Quality is so subjective, but it's easy to count. If you ask heterosexual people how often they have sex, you get the same answer in large parts of the Western world: Heterosexual couples have sex once or twice a week. Cohabiting couples have more sex than married couples. Single people have the least sex.[8] We know less about homosexual men and lesbians, but some data suggest that lesbian couples have around as much sex as heterosexual couples.[9]

Norwegians are no different. In a Norwegian study involving couples aged between twenty-three and sixty-seven, around 40 percent had had sex once or twice a week in the previous month.[10] Only one eager group, 10 percent of the total, had had sex three, four, or more times a week. Just as many hadn't had sex at all in the previous month. The rest had had sex once every other week or less.

In this study there was, perhaps surprisingly, not such a great difference between how often the different age groups had sex. Only when couples hit fifty did they begin to have sex a little less often, but even then, more than 40 percent had sex once or twice a week or more. Even so, we know from a long series of studies that age is one of the most important factors when it comes to how often people in relationships have sex. Among others, this is because the body's sexual functioning deteriorates with age. The libido falls, men get erectile problems, and women may find the mucous membrane in their vaginas becomes fragile and thin due to low estrogen levels, leading to more discomfort during sex. However, there are other factors that explain how often we have sex. One of them is being in love.

The first stage of a new relationship can feel like being in a bubble. The brain is overflowing with neurotransmitters that convey pleasure, satisfaction, and desire. Absorbed in the feeling of being in love, you forget that anything exists apart from the two of you. Sex becomes more important than sleep, food, and friends. It becomes a shared language to convey everything you don't yet dare say with words: It's you and me now—the only thing that matters.

Everyday life has a way of sneaking up on you in the end. One evening, you catch yourself looking at the clock as an eager hand creeps under your underwear. "Can't we just cuddle? I have to get up so early," you say with an apologetic smile. Is there something wrong with your relationship if you're suddenly not so into having sex 24/7? Or is it just a natural development?

A German study examined the sex lives of 1,900 students in their twenties who were in steady relationships.[11] It found a clear connection between how long the couples had been together and how often they had sex. On average, the newly enamored couples had sex ten times a month, or two and a half times a week. Seventy percent had sex more than seven times a month. After the first year, the number of times people had sex began to decrease. When the relationship had lasted between one and three years, fewer than half of respondents had sex two or more times a week. After five years, it hit rock bottom. By then, the frequency of sex was halved, from ten to five times a month. These findings have also been seen in other studies[12, 13] and among lesbian couples.[14]

In other words, you're not alone if you feel like you're having less sex than before, but what's going on here? The German study made some interesting observations. At the beginning of a relationship, women and men experienced similar levels of sexual desire and had the same desire for intimacy and nearness. Then something odd happened. While the men were still just as horny three years later, the study found a dramatic reduction in sexual desire among women after the first year of the relationship had passed. During the first year, three out of four women agreed that they wanted to have sex often. After three years the number had fallen to just one in four. Twice as many as at the beginning, up from 9 percent to 17 percent, said they often experienced a lack of sexual desire.[15]

One illustration of this is how often men and women in a relationship find themselves being rejected when they feel like having sex. In the Norwegian study we spoke about earlier, half the men said they were sexually rejected now and then, while one in ten felt they were often rejected. The number was reversed for women. Ninety percent of the women said they'd never or rarely been sexually rejected by their partner.

One aspect that didn't decrease but rather increased over the course of the relationship was the women's need for intimacy and nearness. For men, however, the desire for cuddling *decreased* over time. Perhaps the cliché is truer than we'd like to believe: women want to cuddle, men want to fuck. Why, we don't know. The researchers behind the German study thought the best explanation was evolutionary. Women unconsciously use sex as a means of binding the man to them and then lose interest in sex once their goal is achieved and the man is embedded in the relationship. Others believe the answer lies in different degrees of biological sex drive (whether or not sexual desire is a drive at all is something we'll come back to later [page 95]). Still others point out that society has so-called sexual scripts for how men and women should behave. People think of having a strong sex drive as manly, whereas it's considered unfeminine for women to express the same degree of desire. This may make it easier for women to settle into asexual patterns than men, but it can also increase the experience of shame in men who have little interest in sex.

So far, we've seen that the longer a couple is together, the less sex they have. At the same time, we know that the happiest couples are the ones who have the most sex. One consolation is that there seems to be a happiness ceiling. A Canadian study of 30,000 people found that the level of happiness didn't increase among people who had sex more than once a week.[16] So it seems that human beings may have found their way to a golden mean of once or twice a week all by themselves!

So which aspects other than frequency are involved in determining how satisfied we are with our sex lives? Again, the answer may seem obvious: the quality of the relationship.[17, 18, 19] There is a close connection between how satisfied we are with our relationship and the quality of our sex life. Put simply, a good sex life is a good relationship. We don't know whether it's the good sex that makes us satisfied with the relationship or the good relationship that produces good sex. It's probably a mixture.

A good relationship has a lot to do with communication. You have to talk to each other about sex and feelings. Oh, God—how lame! Why on earth do we have to talk about sex? Isn't that just the ultimate proof that your relationship is sexually dead? The sexiest thing about one-night stands and new relationships is precisely the lack of talk. People are so afraid of talking that they'd rather forget the condom than risk killing the atmosphere. This little chat is a threat to the fragile state of mystery and excitement.

Even so, it is simply a fact that couples who can achieve emotional intimacy by talking about their feelings, needs, and expectations are more satisfied with both their relationship and their sex life in the long run.[20, 21, 22] By speaking openly about what you want and need sexually, you create security and, in turn, satisfaction. As a bonus, couples who talk about sex aren't just more satisfied, they also have more sex.[23]

There are many things in a relationship that can kill sexual desire: stress, lack of shared quality time, the feeling of not measuring up sexually, a negative self-image, and poor body awareness. If you feel that you and your partner have different sexual needs, you can quickly find yourself in a vicious circle in which one of you is always taking the initiative and the other is often rejecting the advances. It's no fun rejecting someone. You feel guilty because you can't live up to the other person's expectations and you may start to become anxious that they will eventually get tired of it and leave you. The more you worry about these things, the less desire for sex you have. In the end, you avoid even innocent cuddling or kissing for fear it might lead the other person to expect something more.

This is often the underlying dynamic when couples stop having regular sex. It's naïve to think that you can get over this without talking to each other. If more couples had dared to have a talk as soon as they noticed something was off, a lot of their problems could have been avoided. So sit down with your partner, put away your smartphone, and have a real conversation. Perhaps you'll get more and better sex as a result.

Perhaps you think that quantity isn't everything, and we absolutely agree. Having sex twice a week is great, but it's the *content* that matters. What kind of sex do people actually have? Sex can mean so many things, after all. It may involve sucking and licking, vagina or anus. People may come or not come, do it in a double bed, on a sofa, or in a hotel elevator. For some people, routine sex is their mortal enemy: they miss the excitement and unpredictability of their single life or the beginning of their relationship.

An Australian study from 2006 involving 19,000 people looked at which combinations of sex people had last had.[24] The answer they got was that 12 percent had had only vaginal sex. Half had vaginal sex as well as stimulating each other's sex organs with their hands. A third had also had oral sex. Hardly surprisingly, the study found that the more hands and tongue were involved, the more likely the woman was to have achieved orgasm.

There are a lot of expectations attached to the idea of a good sex life. The reality is that a normal sex life is, well, pretty normal. Very few people are at it like rabbits. People get kind of bored as the first crush dissipates and everyday life catches up with their sex lives. A minority go down on their partner every time they have sex. Even so, most are very satisfied. And if you want things to be better, there's only one thing to do: talk to each other.

DESIRE GONE MISSING

Wanting sex is no longer taboo for women. It's almost become an ideal among young people. The notion of perfection involves enjoying sex, initiating sex, and experimenting with sex. But what are you supposed to do if your desire vanishes or never arrives in the first place? That can leave people feeling self-conscious, excluded, and ashamed.

In 2015, Nina had the pleasure of meeting an unusually fascinating woman. Dr. Shirley Zussman, then one hundred years old, is a little hunchbacked lady with full lips and sparkling eyes. She might be said to have had a front-row seat to the sexual revolution. She studied with William Masters and Virginia E. Johnson—renowned for their "discovery" of the female orgasm and the inspiration for the HBO series *Masters of Sex*. Since the 1960s, Zussman has practiced as a sex therapist in New York.

A half-century later, she still treats patients in her office in New York's Upper East Side, with its floral décor and its bookshelves decked with wooden figures in different sexual positions. This gives her a unique overview of the development of sexual problems over time: "Before, my patients used to come to me with orgasm problems—premature ejaculation or the absence of climax—but now it's simply the spark that's missing," she says. People definitely have better sex nowadays than in the 1960s, according to Zussman, but that's no help when they can't bring themselves to do it at all. She blames it on technology and high pressure at work. "The women who come to me are so tired that they'd rather look at those darn iPhones than set aside time for intimacy. We forget to touch each other and look each other in the eyes."

Dr. Zussman may well be right. It sometimes seems as though lack of desire is the new female ailment. A major study from 2013 showed that one in three British women had suffered from an absence of sexual desire in the previous year.[25] Among women in the sixteen to twenty-four age group, one in four reported that they lacked any interest in sex. It makes for sad reading.

So what yardstick are women who suffer a lack of desire measuring themselves against? Since the 1960s, a kind of domino model has been used, involving four stages of sexual response: Desire—Excitement—Orgasm—Resolution. Desire is defined as a wish for sexual activity, including fantasies and thoughts. Desire is a purely mental process: I want to have sex NOW! Excitement, however, is both a feeling of pleasure and a purely physical reaction that involves, among others, an increased supply of blood to the genitals, moistening and expansion of the vagina, a higher pulse rate, higher blood pressure, and more rapid breathing.

Only lately have researchers begun to question this model. Surveys have, in fact, shown that up to one in three women rarely if ever experience sexual desire—i.e., they do not feel "spontaneous desire" as it's called technically. Even so, most of them experience physical excitement and enjoyment of sex. Perhaps that sounds peculiar. Can it really be true that there's something seriously wrong with so many women out there?[26, 27]

DESIRE

EXCITEMENT

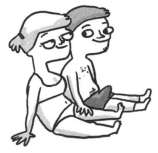

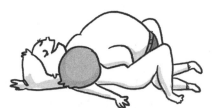

ORGASM

RESOLUTION

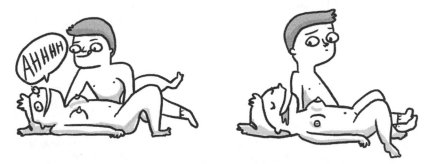

An increasing number of people say no. For many women, desire is actually *responsive*; in other words, it arises precisely as a result of intimate touch or a sexual situation.[28, 29] Physical excitement precedes desire, you might say, and so these women are more dependent on foreplay and nearness to flip the switch. Women with responsive desire have low interest in sex and take little initiative in bed, but they still have the capacity to have great sex once they get going. Desire just has to be encouraged a little more carefully.

The sex researcher Emily Nagoski has taken up the banner of educating women about responsive desire. In her book, *Come as You Are* (2015), she claims that nearly one in three women have a responsive form of sexual desire. At the opposite end of the scale, we find the 15 percent who have the "classic," spontaneous form of sexual desire, in which you feel a desire for sex out of the blue. All the other women are somewhere in between the two.[30] Now and then, they want to have sex without quite understanding why, whereas other times, sex sounds like a drag until they feel their body responding and their head slowly joins the party. Only a small group of around 5 percent lacks any desire for sex, whether spontaneous or responsive.

The model of responsive desire marks a clear divergence from popular culture's presentation of the way sex should be. A lot of girls and women we meet don't recognize themselves in this mainstream image. They wonder if they're abnormal because they're not as interested in sex as "everybody else." They're convinced their boyfriend thinks they're boring, and they feel guilty because they never initiate sex. For a lot of these women, it may be liberating to find out there's another explanatory model. There are plenty of indications that responsive desire is an entirely normal variant of female sexuality and not a flaw or an illness.*

Part of the reason we think spontaneous desire is normal is that it's the dominant form of desire for men. According to Nagoski,

---

* This distinction in types of desire obviously also applies to men, who may experience responsive desire. It's just more rare for this to be a man's primary form of desire. According to Nagoski, around 75 percent of all men primarily experience spontaneous desire versus 15 percent of all women. Five percent of men have responsive desire as their main form versus 30 percent of women.

around three out of four men have the spontaneous type of desire, and for some strange reason we assume that male and female sexuality work the same way. Perhaps they don't, as we'll soon see.

Another source of confusion is the myth that human beings are born with a "sex drive."[31] That we are born with sexual desire. Drives are like instincts that help keep us alive. They are what cause thirst, hunger, and tiredness among others. Our brain sends an unconscious message that it's time to do a particular thing to keep the body in balance, for example sleep, eat, or drink. If we had a sex drive, it would tell us that we have a need for sex along the same lines as our need for food, sleep, and warm clothes. In that case, it would be a need fundamental to our survival. When sex is defined that way, it's not surprising that we think something's seriously wrong with us if we don't experience sexual desire.* And just in case you are in doubt about it: nobody ever died from lack of sex. Sex isn't a drive but a reward.[32]

As long as sex gives enjoyment and is pleasurable, it's like a natural drug for the brain: we want to have more. Desire is stimulated and we begin to seek out situations in which we can get sex. And that's where we come to Nagoski's important point: If sex doesn't serve as a reward for you, e.g., because it's painful, carries associations with earlier assaults, or is just plain boring, your desire diminishes. The system only works as long as sex serves as a reward for the brain. In other words, we're not born with a sexual appetite, we *become* sexually desirous.

We can learn two lessons from this. First of all, it means that women (and men) who have little desire for sex—either generally or because they only experience responsive desire—weren't born abnormal or sick. Some people love chocolate, others don't. We don't think there's anything wrong with people who don't like

---

* Absence or loss of sexual desire is actually a diagnosis in the international classification of mental and behavioral disorders (ICD-10). It is possible to be assigned this diagnosis even if you experience sexual pleasure and arousal. In the American diagnosis system, DSM-V, the equivalent diagnosis has now been changed.

chocolate, even though *most* brains react positively to these delightful combinations of fat and sugar. And incidentally, why does it
matter whether we label people as sick? Well, the tiny remnant of
sexual desire that's left inside is killed stone dead if you're made to
feel like a walking deviant.

Second, the fact that sexual desire is developed implies that it
isn't a constant. We are born with the *potential* to become aroused,
but the extent to which we do so varies over time according to how
much pleasure and satisfaction sex gives us and what our general
life situation is like. In addition, our sexual history—the experiences we've had—helps shape our sexual desire.

Thinking of sexual desire as a reward rather than a drive explains
why it rises and falls in waves over the course of our lives and the
relationships we are involved in. It also gives us a fantastic means of
influencing desire. The brain's system of reward can be manipulated
if we understand how it works. And that brings us to the biggest
difference between men and women.

Sex researchers come up with some very strange ideas. In a raft of
experiments, men and women have had apparatuses attached to
their penises and their vaginas to measure the blood flow to their
sex organs. This is meant to determine how *physically* excited a
person is, but these are automatic responses that people don't consciously control. In the experiments, the subject may watch porn:
hetero sex, homosexual sex, cuddly sex, violent sex, yes, even sex
between apes—something for every taste, in other words. Subjects
then report how aroused they feel as they watch the different clips.
And that's when a very interesting discovery is made.[33, 34]

Among men, there's around a 65 percent correspondence
between how hard their penis is and how aroused they feel, meaning that the brain is mostly on the same page as the automatic
responses of the male sex organ.[35] *Aha, I'm hard, so I must want
sex*, thinks the man. (Of course, this is a simplification. Men can
also become hard without having any desire whatsoever for sex,
as with the well-known phenomenon of "morning wood," or with

teenage boys getting an erection when they have to go up to the blackboard and demonstrate how to do a math problem). Men's desire is pretty closely connected to the shenanigans of the penis, so pills like Viagra work incredibly well when men are struggling to "get it up." Viagra doesn't work on the brain but simply ensures that the veins carrying blood back *out* of the penis become constricted, making the penis grow harder and more engorged with blood. This is more than enough: if you deal with the limitations of the penis, the job's mostly done.

In women, however, it's been found there's only a 25 percent overlap between the brain and the workings of the sex organs.[36] The connection is so minor that it's impossible to say anything at all about how much a woman feels sexual desire based on how wet or engorged her sex organs are. A woman's genitals swell and grow wet from seeing men having sex with men and apes in full swing, but she won't necessarily feel turned on as a result. The women's genitals also responded strongly to lesbian sex, often more than to hetero sex. More disturbingly, it has been observed that women can become physically excited and experience orgasm during sexual assaults.[37] Does this mean that women actually dig ape sex, or that some females like to be raped?

No, no, and no again! It means that women, unlike men, have a much higher degree of what sex researchers call "arousal non-concordance" or "subjective-genital (dis)agreement." These compli-cated terms just mean that there isn't any correspondence between the brain and the nether regions when it comes to desire. The two body parts evidently don't speak the same language, and women with a very low degree of desire score highest of all in terms of non-concordance. Their brains are almost incapable of picking up the signals from their genitals.[38]

Women's desire is first and foremost located in their heads. It's not enough for an attractive person to be lying in our bed or for us to become wet and erect, the way men often do. We need more; it's our brain that needs stimulating, not our genitals. That's why Viagra works on very few women.[39] For women's sexual desire to be affected by pills, you have to fiddle with the intricate pathways in the brain, and *that's* medicine at a whole new level.

Efforts have been made to develop a "pink pill" for women's sexual desire, although they've been largely unsuccessful. One attempt involved giving women testosterone, since this sex hormone is believed to be central to sexual desire. The problem is that it's not a good idea to give testosterone to fertile women due to the potentially damaging effects on a fetus if the woman were to become pregnant. As such, most of the studies were carried out on women who were almost entirely lacking in testosterone either because of cancer surgery or because they'd reached menopause. In these cases, the testosterone boost has mostly been seen to have a moderately positive effect on sexual desire.[40] In the best study, carried out on slightly younger women aged thirty-five to forty-six, no rise in levels of desire was found.[41] However, the women who received a medium-size dose of testosterone experienced an increase of 0.8 in "satisfactory sexual events" in the course of a month compared with the women who received a placebo.

The findings indicate that more testosterone has little effect once a very low minimum level has been exceeded. In fact, studies looking at the effect of testosterone on sexual desire cannot boast any major findings. Whether you're high or low, this doesn't appear to predict where you are on the desire scale.[42] It seems like sex hormones just don't have a very strong influence on women's sexual desire, as had been believed.[43]

Other medication has also been tested. The artificially produced hormone Melanotan, popularly known as the "Barbie drug," which is illegal in the United States, attracted a lot of attention in the Norwegian media at one point because teenage girls, led by Norwegian singer and celebrity blogger Sophie Elise Isachsen, were buying it illegally on the Internet. Melanotan imitates one of the body's hormones that tans our skin and gives us freckles. Melanotan was originally developed to help us tan without sun exposure—in other words as self-tanning in pill form. Then it was discovered that

Melanotan's side effects included reduced appetite (hello, skinny jeans) and, possibly, increased sexual desire. It sounded like mainstream culture's idea of the perfect woman: golden brown and thin, with a big sexual appetite. Understandably enough, the pharma companies saw dollar signs.

But Melanotan use eventually turned out to have potentially life-threatening side effects. All experiments with the drug were halted. Then the pharmaceutical company found that it could produce a less dangerous variant called Bremelanotide. After years of experiments, the medicine is now undergoing a final round of studies and it looks like it will be approved. The problem is that this expensive medicine has to be administered with a syringe, and even then the effect isn't especially impressive. On average, users reported half an extra "satisfying sexual event" *per month* compared with those using a placebo injection.[44] Nothing to write home about.

Another medication, generically known as flibanserin and marketed as Addyi,[45] was originally developed as an antidepressant but was approved in August 2015 for use on premenopausal women diagnosed with low sexual desire. This medication is also incredibly expensive—nearly $1,000 a month[46] if you don't have insurance—and must be used daily. You can't drink alcohol while you're taking it, either, due to the danger of life-threatening drops in blood pressure. Side effects such as nausea, dizziness, and fatigue are relatively common. Here, too, the effects are not dramatic. The users have between 0.4 and one extra "satisfying sexual event" per month.[47]

In other words, pills do not, so far, appear to be the miracle cure for decreased sexual desire that women (and their sexual partners) had been hoping for. None of the medications mentioned here amount to much once you take into account the side effects, price, and effectiveness. However, these kinds of studies have emphasized how much of an impact our feelings have on sexual desire and satisfaction. Indeed, in some of the studies, an incredibly high placebo effect was observed—higher than has been seen for almost any other "medication." In a Viagra study, 40 percent of the women who were given sugar pills were seen to have experienced an increase in sexual desire.[48] By taking a pill, they entered into a new mode and a new role—they managed to break out of old, ingrained patterns in which they had identified themselves as people who didn't want sex.

The placebo effect shows us this: Our sexual desire lives in our head and it can be manipulated. But how?

Emily Nagoski explains it very well.[49] Imagine the brain, holding sway at the top of the body like a sensitive conductor. The body's conductor is constantly receiving signals from the body and its environment, which it interprets, fitting them together to form a finely tuned image. Our nervous system and the signals it sends to the brain are structured very simply, almost like the codes in a computer, where everything is either 0 or 1. We have one signal that tells us to "drive," known as *excitation*, and another that tells us to "brake," or *inhibition*. The balance between the signals indicating excitation and those indicating inhibition determines what the brain will decide to do with the body at any given time. If you're pushing the brake to the floor, it doesn't make any difference if you accelerate at the same time. The end result will be the same: stopping.

Imagine that each of the reasons that prevent you from wanting sex—consciously or unconsciously—puts a little pressure on the brake. Examples could include stress, depression, poor body image, feelings of guilt, and fear of not achieving orgasm. All these slight pressures on the brake build up so that the brake ends up pressed to the floor, bringing things to a complete halt. In order to relieve this heavy pressure on the brake, our brains need to receive an even more powerful signal telling us to drive—for example, love and pleasure. The reward must be greater than the effort. Now and then, this happens by itself, for example, when we're in love; but otherwise, our task is to ensure that the "drive" signals are allowed to dominate and that the brake is as weak as possible. This sounds pretty vague, but there's actually no mystery about it. The first step is acknowledging that sexual desire is not something that arises of its own accord, or a fixed character trait you were born with. After that, you have to think about what turns you off and on. Do what Nagoski says: make a list.

What turns me off? *Having sex right before I go to sleep because then I worry I won't be well rested the next day. Feeling down or sad. Fear that my partner will try to have sex when I don't feel like it and then I'll have to reject him/her again. Uncertainty about the relationship. Jealousy. Routine sex when I know exactly what's going to happen. The expectation that I have to come in order for my partner to feel like a good lover. Stress or worry about things I should have done but didn't get around to during the day. Feeling ugly. When I haven't showered and feel dirty. When we check our cell phones in bed.*

What turns me on? *Knowing that we have lots of time and there's no hurry to get things finished. A quickie, no talking. The thought of an orgasm. Feeling good in my own body. An erotic book or film, or just porn. Sex after exercise, when the endorphins are flowing and the blood's still pumping. Sex in the middle of the day in broad daylight. Pitch-black, sheltering darkness. Clean sheets. Feeling loved. Compliments. New surroundings. Safe surroundings. Seeing my partner in his or her element. Being in my element. Having my back tickled. Daring to try new things in bed. When I'm sure that what I do in bed is the best thing my partner can imagine.*

Once you've written your own list, the real work can begin. You have to arrange things so that the balance tips in favor of "drive." That means eliminating as many of the brakes as possible, while simultaneously creating a setting in which as many of your switches as possible are flipped.

It's pretty much impossible to do this alone if you're in a relationship. You have to involve your partner and tell her or him what turns you on and what you need. In relationships that have gotten stuck in a rut, sex therapists often recommend you stop having sex at all for a while, or establish guidelines for sex—for example, deciding on a particular day and time when you'll have sex and clearing your schedule accordingly. It sounds pretty unsexy, but there's a logic to it. By removing all expectations of sex, you get to have a break until the desire returns of its own accord. You can't force desire. The sense that you *should* be feeling desire is just another brake.

This doesn't mean that you should stop being close to your partner. For a lot of people, in fact, it works the opposite way, because they have space to cuddle and be intimate without feeling any pressure for anything they're not ready for. Be kind to yourself, and patient, too. If your partner doesn't think this is important, perhaps you've discovered the root of the problem.

Dr. Zussman, with her hundred years of experience, has grasped something vital. Sexual desire doesn't occur in a vacuum. Desire is tightly interwoven with our relationships, including our relationship with ourselves. There are no quick fixes, but most of us are capable of feeling desire.

THE BIG O

The orgasm is a wonderful, fabulous phenomenon. It stands apart from all the tedious routine work the body does to keep us alive. While the heart beats to pump blood around our bodies, the gut rumbles and churns to give us nourishment, and the brain quivers with nerve signals to move our body and make plans, the orgasm has a completely unique function. The orgasm is quite simply toe-curling, hair-raising, moaning bliss. The orgasm is our little reward.

People have tried to come up with many different definitions of what orgasms actually are, and researchers aren't entirely in agreement about it. The traditional medical understanding of it is that the orgasm is a transient peak sensation of intense sexual pleasure, associated with rhythmic contractions of the musculature in the pelvic region.[50]

Modern sex researchers think this definition is too narrow. Orgasms are experienced differently from one woman to another; what's more, it's physically possible to experience unpleasant orgasms or asexual orgasms—for example, during an assault or while asleep. In fact, as many as one in three women experience orgasms in their sleep.[51] Some researchers therefore think it's better to say that orgasms are a sudden, involuntary release of sexual tension,[52] like the release of a tensed bow.

We know that people can have orgasms without pleasure, orgasms without physical contact with the genitals, and orgasms without circumvaginal contractions. Some describe just having a warm, tingling feeling that spreads throughout their whole body, and then getting an unmistakable feeling of being "finished." Common to all is that you know it when you've had an orgasm. If you don't know whether you've had an orgasm, you haven't had one. It's so vague, and yet so simple.

If we stick to the classic concept of the orgasm, the orgasm is the peak of sexual response. When women are physically excited, their inner labia and the inner parts of their clitoris fill with blood, in the same way as a man's penis becomes hard. In fact, the clitoral complex doubles in size when you're aroused! Just ten to thirty seconds after stimulation of the genitals has begun, the vagina will, often as not, start to become wet. It will also become at least a centimeter broader and longer. The closer you come to climax, the more your pulse quickens, your breathing speeds up, and your blood pressure climbs. Many people also feel the muscles in the rest of their body tensing, with their fingers and toes curling against whatever surface they're on. There's a wonderful name for this: carpopedal spasms.

In the end, the orgasm arrives. A feeling of well-being spreads through you from head to toe. It feels as if your genitals are exploding, and the muscles in your pelvic region will often tighten in rhythmic contractions. The contractions start in the lower part of the vagina and spread upward to embrace the whole of the vagina and the uterus. The muscles around your urethra and anus are often involved, too. On average, women's orgasms last around seventeen seconds.[53] When you're finished, however, the blood will begin to withdraw from the genitals, in the same way that a man's penis becomes flaccid after orgasm. At that point the body has completed the resolution phase—where everything slowly returns to its normal state.

Unlike men, women can have several orgasms in a row if they continue to stimulate themselves. The world record for the number of female orgasms is unknown. For some reason or another, the Guinness Book of World Records hasn't published it, although other wickedly exciting sex records such as "most frequent sex" are available on its website. In case you were wondering, the Ornebius aperta cricket from Australia is the record holder, with fifty sex acts in the course of three to four hours. The rascal!

The highest unofficial figure we know of for number of orgasms is from a so-called Masturbate-a-Thon—which is, marvelously, a self-pleasuring competition to raise money for charity.[54] The record is from the Danish Masturbate-a-Thon in 2009, in which the winner is supposed to have had a total of 222 orgasms in the course of one, presumably pretty long, masturbation session. That leaves most of us with something to aim for . . .

Now, perhaps you're surprised we're talking about orgasms without specifying what kind, because after all there are clitoral orgasms, vaginal orgasms, G-spot orgasms, tantric orgasms, squirting orgasms, and orgasms from having your toes sucked. Aren't there?

Actually, all orgasms are the same. The physical and mental response is the same. The only difference is what releases it. Our entire body is an erogenous zone. There are nerve endings everywhere that can be stimulated and give pleasure. Just think how delicious it can be to have someone kiss your neck, tickle your scalp, or stroke the inside of your thigh. We've also met women who have spontaneous orgasms throughout the day, every single day, without any kind of physical stimulation, as well as women who can breathe their way to orgasm.

The terms *vaginal orgasm* and *clitoral orgasm* are especially widespread, although there isn't actually any difference between them.[55] We now know that the clitoris is a large organ and not just a little nub at the front of the vulva. The inner parts of the clitoris surround both the urethra and the vagina, and they can be indirectly stimulated through the vulva and vagina. To talk about clitoral orgasm and vaginal orgasm is imprecise, since the clitoris is thoroughly involved in vaginal sex. The vagina itself is pretty insensitive. As you'll see later, the head of the clitoris is also placed differently for different women. Some people claim that this placement can make it harder or easier for women to achieve orgasm during vaginal intercourse.[56]

Squirting orgasm, female ejaculation, or simply "squirting" is veiled in legend and has been described in literature for more than two thousand years, ever since the time of Aristotle.[57] For most women, however, the urethra isn't especially involved in their sex life, despite being positioned between the head of the clitoris and the vagina. That said, some women find that something special happens with their urethra when they orgasm—a cause of much head scratching among the women themselves as well as researchers. When these women come, clear or milk-white fluid squirts out of their urinary opening. Some women report several milliliters of liquid, while others talk about an amount equivalent to a full glass of milk. What kind of orgasm is *that*?

We don't know how many women have squirting orgasms, but we do know that it happens, and lots of us have seen it on the Internet. Porn depicting ejaculating women was banned in the United Kingdom in 2014 (along with a number of other sex acts that were absurdly deemed potentially harmful, like spanking and facesitting).[58] We don't know why female ejaculation is worse than other porn, for example, porn involving male ejaculation, but it seems that some people find female ejaculation especially offensive, perhaps because they think the ejaculate is urine. But is it?

It's still unclear what the fluid consists of. Some studies argue that the ejaculate comes from some small glands known as Skene's glands. These glands are in the anterior wall of the vagina, around the lower part of the urethra. Apparently not all women have them, and they can vary in size from one woman to the next—which could explain why only some women have squirting orgasms. According to this view, the glands are the equivalent of a man's prostate, which is involved in producing the fluid in sperm, and they empty their secretions into the urethra during orgasm.[59, 60] This theory is supported by the fact that prostate substances have been found in the fluid from some ejaculating women.[61] However, one study from 2015, which used ultrasound examinations on seven masturbating women, concluded that the ejaculate mostly consisted of urine, although small amounts of prostate substances were also found in the liquid.[62] Some researchers think we're dealing with two different phenomena: some women ejaculate small amounts of white fluid from their Skene's glands, while others squirt larger amounts of clear liquid from their bladder.[63] In any case, perhaps it doesn't really matter what the secretion consists of. It's a natural part of orgasm for a number of women.

Let's go back to the story of clitoral and vaginal orgasms. Women have long struggled with a sense that there's a hierarchy of orgasms, with the so-called vaginal orgasm, triggered solely by vaginal penetration, at the top. They feel like there's something wrong with them if they don't get orgasms from nothing but "the old in-out," as Alex DeLarge in *A Clockwork Orange* (1962) likes to call it, or that they're cheating if they have to help things along with a finger or a tongue in order to come.

This is peculiar. Not just because an orgasm is an orgasm whichever way you look at it, but also because reaching orgasm without clitoral stimulation is unusual for most women. How has this strange ranking of female orgasms come about?* Whatever it is, it's a thoroughly modern concept, *not* a leftover from the olden days. Before the times of the Enlightenment people believed a woman had to have an orgasm in order to become pregnant.[64] And if you really wanted to ensure pregnancy, a man and woman supposedly had to come *simultaneously*. In those days, with high infant

---

*   The following historical account is inspired by Liv Strömquist's fantastic graphic novel, *Kunskapens frukt* (Galago, 2014).

mortality rates, having plenty of children was an important goal. Giving women orgasms therefore became an art men had to perfect if they wanted to make sure they had heirs. The key to the woman's orgasm lay in direct stimulation of the head of the clitoris.

Thus the physician to the princess of Austria recommended in 1740 that "the vulva of Her Most Holy Majesty should be titillated before intercourse."[65] Doctors these days could draw some inspiration from this. Imagine if instead of being told to live healthier, you were told you ought to get your lady parts titillated more often. Now that's what we call healthy living!

The men of the 1700s knew the lay of the land even though they misunderstood a lot of other things here on Earth. The source of the inferiority complex surrounding the so-called clitoral orgasm lies a lot closer to our own times. Let's take a trip to the 1900s.

The distinction between vaginal and clitoral orgasms and the elevation of the vaginal as the "true" orgasm is a modern, male invention. Sigmund Freud, the father of psychoanalysis, proposed a new theory in 1905[66] that viewed the clitoral orgasm as the immature young woman's form of orgasm. It was the kind of thing that should only happen in a little girl's bedroom. As soon as the girl got a sniff of a male member, her interest in the clitoris should vanish and be replaced by a burning desire for penetration. The fusion of man and woman was the only healthy form of sex, and the only form that should give women pleasure. Real women, according to Freud, had vaginal orgasms.[67]

Where did Freud get this from? His own head, of course! It didn't matter that there were a bunch of women out there who profoundly disagreed with him. Because they, according to Freud, were ill. These women were suffering from a vaguely defined condition known as frigidity, characterized first and foremost by the fact that they were unable to take pleasure from a man's penis the way they should. It was the ultimate manipulation technique: either you agreed with Freud or you were crazy.[68]

According to Freud, women should seek immediate help from a psychologist if they thought it was wonderful to touch their clitoris or—heaven forbid—failed to have orgasms during vaginal intercourse with their husband. Of course, this was great for men. If a woman didn't come, it wasn't his qualities as a lover that were in question but the woman who needed to do some work on herself. Men had now been given official permission to go for it, come, and then happily turn his back as he switched off the light. A woman's pleasure was her own responsibility.

Freud was hardly a nobody, and his theory gained plenty of support. And that's how thousands of years of female experience were suddenly written off as maidenly neuroses. The clitoris, known for centuries as the core of female sexual pleasure, was consigned to oblivion and vanished from the anatomy books. It would be nearly sixty years before anybody dared contradict Freud's theory.

In the 1960s, a quiet revolution began to take shape at Washington University Hospital, in St. Louis. The gynecologist William Masters and his research partner, Virginia E. Johnson, began to develop an interest in female sexuality and set up a series of experiments that were pretty unconventional. They recruited couples to have sex in the laboratory, hooking them up to measuring equipment and keeping them under observation. They even made a vibrating plastic penis with a camera in its tip so that they could observe what was happening inside a woman's vagina when she came. The result of their studies was seen as a shocking medical discovery: The clitoris was absolutely central to the female orgasm. A bombshell? Obviously.

Today, we know that fewer than a third of all women regularly come from vaginal intercourse alone, and even then, there's much to suggest that the clitoris is central to their orgasm. Some researchers think these women drew the golden ticket in the anatomical lottery, because it seems they have a particular advantage when it comes to the size and placement of their clitoris. The first person to conduct scientific research in this area was another princess, Marie Bonaparte of France, who—despite her great appetite for sex and lovers—was never satisfied because she couldn't come vaginally.[69] Bonaparte and modern researchers both agree on one thing: a larger clitoris head combined with a shorter distance between the clitoris and the vagina makes it easier to have orgasms,[70, 71] because the clitoris enjoys a greater degree of indirect stimulation during penetration, both externally and toward the inner parts of the clitoris. Bonaparte took the drastic step of opting to have her clitoris moved farther down by surgery—unfortunately with poor results.[72]

We wish Bonaparte had known that not having an orgasm during ordinary intercourse with a man isn't abnormal. It's the norm. But because men have dominated the research into female sexuality and the public discourse about sex, this is a message that has passed many people by. Sex has become synonymous with the activity that almost solely ensures that the man comes: the penis in the vagina. Indeed, people say that intercourse isn't "consummated" unless the man has had an orgasm. If only the woman comes, intercourse is theoretically incomplete—it is interrupted intercourse. The woman has vanished from the picture.

The sex you have regularly should be designed to maximize pleasure and orgasms for both partners, so couldn't having sex in a hetero relationship just as well mean, for example, fifty-fifty oral sex and penetration? It's wrong to write off the female orgasm as a pure bonus. Orgasm should be the rule, for women as well as men.

Still, there's no getting away from the fact that it's more difficult for women to have orgasms than men. The proportion of women who are anorgasmic—i.e., they've *never* had an orgasm, either alone or with another person—is between 5 and 10 percent.[73] For men, the opposite most often applies: they struggle with coming too quickly. A major British study found that 21 percent of women aged sixteen to twenty-four found it difficult to have orgasms during sex.[74] Most women find themselves in the "comes now and then" category.

Some fortunate women don't know what we're talking about. We all have one of those irritating friends who tells us that she *always* comes, and usually three or four times every time she has sex. What's the magic trick, you ask? Unfortunately, chances are she won't be able to help you. Although, of course, magic tricks may make a small contribution, there are also real differences between us in terms of how easily we come, and there's nothing we can do about it. These differences are determined, among others, by our genes. Very few of us like to think about our parents having sex, but it's not unlikely that their sex life is a bit reminiscent of your own. If you're an orgasm queen, perhaps you should thank your mom and dad.

Researchers who study twins have found that our genes can explain up to a third of the variation in how often people have orgasms during sex.[75, 76] Perhaps that doesn't sound like a lot, but in the context of genetics, it's nothing to scoff at. Researchers have also looked at frequency of orgasm during masturbation, and here heredity plays an even more important role. In fact, studies show that our genes explain half of the variation in masturbatory orgasms. At first it may seem peculiar that there's a difference between how far genes influence sex and masturbation, respectively; however, masturbation can be thought of as a more genuine reflection of your physical capacity for orgasm, since you're eliminating the psychological uncertainty and sexual interplay that comes with partnered sex.

Another thing that has a major influence on women's capacity to have orgasms is the context in which they have sex. Most women have little chance of reaching orgasm during a one-night stand. American college students responded that only one in ten had an orgasm the first time they slept with a new partner, whereas almost 70 percent of the women had an orgasm when they'd been in a relationship for more than six months.[77]

So there are hereditary differences when it comes to how easily we have orgasms, but the encouraging news is that most women can have orgasms if they want to. The challenge is taking the step from having orgasms alone or now and then, to having them almost always. We aren't saying it's easy, or that it's necessary to stress about how often you have an orgasm, but we are saying it's possible if you're willing to work on it. Here is our orgasm bible, inspired by the advice that women who can't achieve orgasm are often given in therapy.

ORGASM BIBLE

1. **Practice makes perfect.** If you've never masturbated before, it's time to put it on your calendar, literally. Masturbation is a worthwhile use of your time.[78] In studies of women who have never had orgasms, between 60 and 90 percent managed to achieve orgasm, both alone and with a partner, after five or six weeks of regular training.[79] We promise that it's the most fun form of exercise a doctor can recommend. Use your fingers or buy yourself a vibrator. Do whatever turns you on and gets you into the right mood. Do you prefer erotic literature, do you like porn, or do you want to fantasize? The most important thing is that you must NOT start out thinking about an orgasm as a goal, but rather focus on finding techniques you like and that make you feel good. Practice feeling your way toward pleasure and opening yourself up to it. Practice emptying your head of all disturbing thoughts, whether it's the extra rolls of fat on your stomach or that looming exam. The better you get at giving yourself orgasms, the greater the likelihood that you'll have them when you're with a partner. Remember, too, that it's never wrong to take matters into your own hands when you're with a partner. Who does what isn't so important, as long as you're having a good and satisfying time together.

2. **Demand your rights.** Your partner must be included in Project Orgasm. It's important here not to step on anybody's toes—make it a pleasurable joint project. It isn't your partner's fault that you're not coming, unless he or she downright refuses to make any effort to satisfy you. In fact, you have to do the prep work. Your genitals don't come with a user manual, so without your guidance, your partner could spend a year and a day figuring out how to make you come.

The simplest thing is to do the job yourself at the outset, by touching yourself while you have intercourse or by masturbating together. After a while you can teach your partner your tricks. A lot of people find this embarrassing, but it's the only way to do it. Don't expect to get it right the first time. Be patient and praise your partner every time he or she does something that works, that way you'll gradually train a super lover.

3. **Teach yourself the CAT position.** There are many sexual positions and, as you've now learned, few of them are especially suited to giving women orgasms. However, one sexual position has a special status: the CAT position. It's been shown that a variant of the missionary position known as coital alignment technique, or CAT, is especially good for giving women orgasms.[80, 81] This is a position that requires a little practice and coordination, but it repays your patience, in all respects.

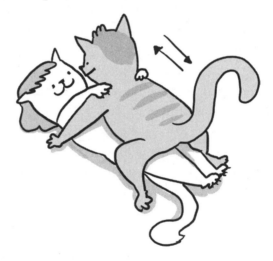

In the CAT position, instead of resting on his hands, your partner must rest on his lower arms and keep as much of his body as possible in contact with yours. Instead of the usual in-and-out thrusting, he should slide his body up along yours horizontally until his genitals are lying right on top of yours. At the same time, you should press your crotches together, like a wave crashing against the shore (clichéd, but true). His hips should tip downward so that his pubic bone and the root of his penis rub against your clitoris. You'll be able to tell when he's doing it right. You should keep your legs as straight and closed as possible; try wrapping your legs around his so that your ankles are resting on the back of his calves.

Whereas the regular missionary position involves humping, the CAT position is based on good old-fashioned rubbing. The penis won't go very deep into your vagina, but will instead give maximum stimulation to the outer couple of centimeters where most of the nerve endings are located; at the same time, your clitoris will receive constant contact.

Once you've got the hang of it, you can try reverse CAT, where you lie on top. Then you have full control and can adjust your clitoral stimulation to exactly the tempo and pressure you want.

4. **Don't relax!** "Relax, relax," you're often told. This may be the world's best and worst advice. Yes, you should try to relax in your head, but if you lie there motionless and expect the orgasm to hit you like a bolt of lightning, you're on the wrong track. It's a matter of tightening up your body. Clench your buttocks together and try to tense the muscles in your genitals, preferably tightening and relaxing them, as if in an orgasmic rhythm or in time with your breathing.

For one thing, this increases the blood flow to your genitals—in other words, you turn yourself on. For another, it's a kind of mental exercise in directing your attention to where the action is. You can try, but it's really hard to think about the pizza you'll be having for dinner at the same time you're working to clench all your pelvic muscles.

At the beginning, it can be difficult to make contact with these muscles. After all, there isn't a "Shape Up—Vagina Edition" available at your local gym. But there ought to be. Lots of women who do regular pelvic floor exercises find they have stronger and easier orgasms. In addition, this prevents urine leaks and pelvic organ prolapse, and may help combat pain during sex.[82] You can do your pelvic floor exercises anywhere—on the bus or before going to bed. You can also use vaginal balls, although that's absolutely not necessary.

5. **Go for a run.** Exercise, especially right before sex, makes it easier for you to get aroused and increases many people's capacity to reach orgasm.[83]

6. **Put on some socks.** This advice is both jokey and serious. The point is that our brain is continually getting signals from the body about how we're feeling. These signals, and the thoughts they provoke, compete for our attention. It's difficult to have an orgasm when your mind is on all sorts of things other than what's going on in your genitals—for example, the fact that your feet are cold. We women are especially prone to these kinds of distractions. The sex researcher Alfred Kinsey observed that female rats, unlike male rats, were easily distracted by tempting crumbs of cheese during the sex act.[84]

The lesson here (it's one that most women tend to forget) is that you have to do everything you can to create the conditions in which it's possible to focus all your attention on having a sizzling time. If that means all the lights have to be switched off, that you want to have sex with your T-shirt on, or, yes, that you have to put on a pair of socks, listen to that inner voice. Be kind to yourself. Orgasms only come when you feel comfortable enough, both physically and mentally, that you can shut everything else out.

PART 4: CONTRACEPTION

When a woman and a man have sex, it can result in a pregnancy. This won't come as a shock to anyone. Sex is fab, and most people want to have sex more times than the number of children they plan to have. If you're heterosexual and want to have vaginal sex without getting pregnant, you're going to have to use some form of contraception.

By *contraception*, we are referring to all methods that can reduce the risk of sexual intercourse leading to pregnancy. In other words, coitus interruptus, also known as withdrawal, is a method of contraception—although it's not one we recommend.

Contraception is hardly a new invention, but as the medical profession has developed, more sophisticated methods have come onto the market. Still, many of the current forms of contraception have a long history. There's nothing new about condoms, but they used to be made of animal hide rather than latex. Four thousand years ago in ancient Greece, women are said to have put a mixture of honey and leaves in their vaginas to keep sperm cells out of the uterus. This is reminiscent of the modern-day diaphragm, a plastic disk that is placed over the cervix to bar the way of sperm cells. Although the diaphragm hasn't been used much in Norway for a long time now, it is sometimes used in other countries, including the United States, where it's available by prescription only. In other countries, such as Sweden, its popularity may be due to an antihormone trend. Clearly, contraception is also a matter of fashion. Withdrawal is hardly a new discovery: There's even a story about it in Genesis (about a guy called Onan), and you can be sure that a couple somewhere will be doing just that this evening. Or right now.

We humans have actually given most things a try, but the advantage we have today is the opportunity to choose. We have plenty of tried-and-tested alternatives that we know work well. If avoiding pregnancy is your goal, it's important to find a reliable method that suits you, your health, and your lifestyle.

Often taken for granted, contraception really is incredible. It gives you the option to choose whether you want to have children at all without this choice affecting your sex life. If you want to have children, you can choose when, with whom, and how many children there will be. Withdrawal, the diaphragm, and a combination of plants and honey in the vagina probably had a certain effect, but the big difference came with the development of the contraceptive pill in the 1950s.[1]

The 1960 debut of the Pill ignited a revolution. The Pill was an effective means of contraception then and it's even better today. The Pill changed women's ability to choose what kind of relationship to be in. They could control their own sex lives and plan their family to suit their career and economic situation. Since its introduction, many new forms of contraception have been developed, including long-acting methods such as the contraceptive implant and the hormonal intrauterine device (IUD), which are our top recommendations.

After that historical background, it's time to talk about the situation today. To be honest, the facts about contraception are dry, very dry. We've done our best to explain the difference between the various methods of contraception, including how to use them, and some tips and tricks as a bonus. But it's all very technical. Consequently, our contraception discussion will probably be the most boring part of the book for some of you—but stick with it. It's probably the most important topic we write about.

We know what young women are wondering about when it comes to contraception because of the many complex questions they've asked us. That's hardly surprising because contraception is a complicated business that all women, for some reason, are expected to understand intuitively, almost without guidance. We also know that an incredible number of myths about contraception persist and

Combined contraceptives with estrogen and progestin	Progestin contraception With progestin, without estrogen	Hormone-free contraception	Emergency contraception
Pill	Contraceptive injection	Condom	Copper IUD
Contraceptive patch	Contraceptive implant	Copper intra-uterine device (IUD)	Pill 1 Levonorgestrel (Norlevo™, Plan B, One-Step)
Vaginal ring	Hormonal intra-uterine device (IUD)	Calendar Method or Fertility Awareness Method	Pill 2: Ulipristal acetate (ELLAONE™, ella)
	Mini pill		
	Estrogen-free mini pill		

that many people suffer unnecessary side effects due to incorrect use, or feel uncertain because they don't have enough information. We don't know whether this is because health professionals who prescribe contraception are providing bad or too little information or because it's all too much to take in at once.

Our aim in this chapter is to give you a basic introduction to contraception so that you have the means to choose a method for yourself. Contraception is in a constant process of development and we recommend that you not only seek out and listen to the advice of health professionals, who may have newer and more detailed knowledge of the contraceptive methods you're interested in, but also don't hesitate to ask your providers questions after you start using a new method of contraception.

HORMONAL CONTRACEPTION

What is it about hormonal contraception that prevents pregnancy? What exactly is going into your system when you swallow your contraceptive pill every morning, insert your vaginal ring every third week, or get a contraceptive implant put in your arm?

Hormonal contraception contains an extremely low dose of the same hormones that are produced in the ovaries and that are involved in controlling the menstrual cycle. All types of hormonal contraception contain something called progestin. This is a synthetic version of the progesterone produced by the body. Some contraceptive methods also include estrogen. These are known as combined contraceptives, while those that only contain progestin are called progestin-only products.

HORMONAL CONTRACEPTION WITH ESTROGEN

There are three types of combined contraceptives: the combined pill, the vaginal ring, and the contraceptive patch. The advantage of combined contraceptives is that the estrogen gives you the option to control your bleeding. The disadvantage is that not everybody can use estrogen, which you'll read more about later (page 166).

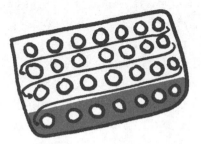

The *combined pill* is the most commonly used combined contraceptive, and there are many types, all of which are slightly different. First of all, different types of estrogen and progestin are used. Second, different combined pills have different dosages of progestin and estrogen. Both of these aspects can affect what side effects you experience, both positive and negative, but you can't know in advance how the particular type of combined pill will work for you. It's a matter of trial and error until you find the brand that suits you.

There are two main categories of combined pill: multiphasic and monophasic. But what on earth does this mean? Most pills are monophasic. If you use this type, it doesn't matter where you start in the blister pack, because the hormone dose is the same in every pill. In other words, all the hormone pills in the pack are identical. Most monophasic pills are designed so that you can, in a way, create an artificial menstrual cycle consisting of a given number of days. Most types involve a twenty-eight-day cycle. So you take hormone pills for twenty-one days of the cycle and during these days, you won't have any bleeding. The last seven days are the so-called pill-free week. Then you can either take the sugar pills included in some packs or take a break from the pills. During these hormone-free days, the endometrium is usually expelled by the uterus, so you'll have bleeding. Examples of monophasic pills that use the twenty-one plus seven days design are Loestrin and Yasmin. Some monophasic pills are organized so that you take twenty-four pills in a row, and then take a break from the hormone pills for four days. Examples of combined pills that use the twenty-four plus four days design are Yaz and Zoely. If you don't want any bleeding at all, you can go on directly to a new pack of hormone pills without taking a break. More about that later (page 152).

Multiphasic pills don't have the same dose of hormones in every pill, and each brand has its own cycle design when it comes to the number of days of hormone pills and the number of days of bleeding. So you can't start at any point in the pack with multiphasic pills: you have to follow the instructions carefully. If you use multiphasic pills, it's extra important to read the patient information leaflet to use them properly, especially if you're planning to skip your periods. Multiphasic pills currently sold in the United States include Ortho-Novum, Necon, Ortho Tri-Cyclen, and Natazia.

When you use combined pills, you're protected against pregnancy the whole time, even on the days when you don't take hormone pills. So you can have sex whenever you want without having to use additional contraception to prevent pregnancy. But if you miss your pill, you may lose that protection. How many pills you can miss before there's a chance of becoming pregnant depends on the type of pill, so refer to the patient information leaflet and instructions from your doctor. When missed pills lead to poor protection against pregnancy, we call it contraceptive failure.[2]

The *vaginal ring* is a plastic ring you insert into your vagina. It looks like a soft, round, spaghetti-thin doughnut. In the United States, only one type is currently sold, NuvaRing. To insert it into your vagina, you simply press it together with two fingers and push it far in. When you release your grip on it, the ring will spring back into its original shape, adjusting to the inner walls of the vagina and holding itself in place. To remove it, just fish it out gently with your middle finger.

The vaginal ring also contains a combination of estrogen and progestin. The hormones pass through the mucous membranes in the vagina and end up in the bloodstream. A lot of people think it sounds unpleasant to walk around with something in their vaginas. They also wonder if the ring can get lost inside them.

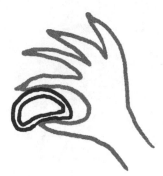

Once you've inserted the ring, you shouldn't notice it's there—just like with a tampon. But watch out! Although it isn't common, there have been cases of vaginal rings falling out and ending up in the toilet. This happened to one of our female friends when she was out on the town late one night. She told us she didn't notice it was gone until the next afternoon. When you're drinking alcohol, it's easy to become a bit less aware of what's going on. It's a good idea to get into the habit of sticking a finger in your vagina now and then to check that the ring's in place.

As with most monophasic pills, you should use the ring for twenty-one consecutive days, i.e., three weeks in a row. You can use the same ring for three weeks before taking a seven-day break for bleeding. You can also put a new ring in immediately, without a break, if you want to skip the bleeding.

Although you won't notice the ring is there, your partner may feel it when you have vaginal sex. Some women prefer to take it out before sex, which is perfectly safe to do. It's okay to take the ring out for three hours at a time, but it's important to remember to put it back in again after the three hours, otherwise you'll lose your protection against pregnancy.[3]

The *hormonal patch* is placed directly on the skin, and the hormones pass through your skin and into your bloodstream. The patch sold in the United States is called Ortho Evra. You can use each patch for a week and, as with the ring and most monophasic pills, you should receive hormones for twenty-one days in a row. You use

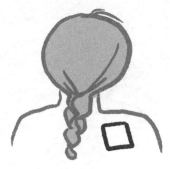

three patches, one per week, before taking a seven-day break. If you forget to change the patch in time or if it comes loose, contraceptive failure may occur.[4]

HOW DO COMBINED CONTRACEPTIVES PREVENT PREGNANCY?

It may seem odd that hormones we already have in our body can prevent pregnancy, but the progestin and estrogen in the combined products work extremely well.

What the main combined contraceptives do is prevent the ovulation that occurs once in every menstrual cycle—roughly once a month. As we discussed earlier, if you have unprotected sex from around five days before ovulation, including the day you ovulate, you may become pregnant. This period is called the fertile window.

You could say that the usage of hormonal contraception tricks the body into believing that you are pregnant. When you're pregnant, your menstrual cycle comes to a halt, as if somebody pressed the Pause button. If your menstrual cycle stops, there's no ovulation, and without ovulation there's no fertile window or possibility of fertilization.

The progesterone that is naturally produced in the body is responsible for this pause when you become pregnant. Progesterone tells the pituitary gland in the brain not to produce the FSH and LH hormones anymore—hormones that are necessary to keep the menstrual cycle going. There's no follicular phase without FSH and no ovulation without LH.

The progestin in hormonal contraception does the same thing as progesterone does in the body when you become pregnant. Progestin tells the brain it's time to stop the menstrual cycle for a while. In a way, you could say that combined contraceptives trick the body into thinking it's already pregnant.

Combined contraceptives prevent pregnancy in several ways—they don't just stop ovulation. After sexual intercourse, sperm cells must swim up through the cervix and into the uterus. The progestin in combined contraceptives makes the mucus in the cervix thicker so that it's more difficult for the sperm cells to swim into the uterus. In addition, the endometrium becomes thinner than usual. This makes it difficult for fertilized eggs to fasten themselves onto the uterine lining.

Estrogen is usually responsible for growth in the uterine lining or endometrium, and this lining is what later becomes your period. The estrogen in combined contraceptives makes the endometrium grow a little each month, so most women using combined contraceptives will also have menstruation-like bleeding when they take a short break, of seven days or fewer, from hormones.

ESTROGEN-FREE CONTRACEPTION

The advantage of estrogen-free contraception is that it can be used by anybody, including women who can't take estrogen for one reason or another. In the United States, physicians and health care providers recommend contraception based on a woman's age, lifestyle, medical and sexual history, and insurance coverage. Long-acting contraceptive methods, such as the hormonal IUD and the contraceptive implant, are both estrogen-free and are the methods that offer the most effective protection against pregnancy. While the Norwegian health authorities recommend them as first choice, these options may be cost-prohibitive depending on where you are and your type of health coverage. The disadvantage with estrogen-free contraception is that you may not have such good control over bleeding as with combined contraceptives. In other words, you can't decide when you'll have your period if you use estrogen-free contraception. Usually, though, the bleeding is much less heavy than normal when using all forms of hormonal contraception. Our impression is that some women who use the contraceptive implant have problems with persistent bleeding abnormalities, and that this is less of a problem for women using the hormonal IUD. Again, success is a matter of trial and error.

The *contraceptive implant* is a small plastic rod containing progestin. The brand sold in the United States is Nexplanon. It is placed under the skin on the upper arm using a type of syringe and can remain there for three years. It continuously releases a little hormone so that the amount in the blood is constant and low. The contraceptive implant is the safest contraceptive method on the market today. Once it's in place on your arm, you can't go wrong. The progestin in the implant will stop your menstrual cycle, allowing you to avoid ovulation as long as it's in your arm.[5]

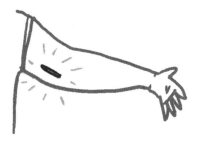

The *hormonal IUD* is a small, T-shaped object that is inserted in the uterus by a trained health professional. It releases a low dose that primarily works locally, in the genital area, although small quantities also pass through the mucous membrane in the uterus and are absorbed into the bloodstream. The dosage of hormone circulating in the bloodstream will be extremely low, and a lot of people who've experienced side effects with other contraceptive methods may therefore suffer fewer problems by switching to the hormonal IUD. You can keep the hormonal IUD in for between three and five years, depending on which type you choose. There are currently three types on the market in Norway and five in the United States. Two that are available in both countries are Mirena and Kyleena. Mirena, which lasts for five years, is the hormonal IUD with the highest dose of hormones and is therefore particularly suitable for women who are interested in having light bleeding. A lot of women find that their periods stop entirely with Mirena. Kyleena, which also lasts for five years, is specially designed for women who haven't given birth. It's smaller than Mirena and has a lower dose of hormones. Even though Kyleena is particularly marketed to women who haven't give birth, it's perfectly fine for younger women to use Mirena, too. Kyleena is a bit larger and some may find the insertion more unpleasant. Mirena gives you better control over your bleeding than with the lower-dose hormonal IUDs and is still a much lower dose of hormone overall than with other methods of contraception. It's just a myth that the hormonal IUD is only suitable for women who've given birth!

Some, but not all, women may find they stop ovulating when they have a hormonal IUD. This is temporary, of course, and depends on the dose of hormones in the IUD. It is more common to stop ovulating when you use the Mirena, since it has a slightly higher hormone dose. Kyleena often contains doses of progestin that are too low to influence the pituitary gland in the brain, but that doesn't mean it doesn't work well. The most important effect of the hormonal IUD is, in fact, local: the progestin makes the mucus in the cervix impenetrable to sperm cells. At the same time, the uterine lining becomes thin, making it difficult for any fertilized eggs to survive there.[6]

All types of hormonal IUDs offer good contraceptive alternatives, providing long-acting, reliable protection against pregnancy. Most women will experience lighter bleeding and less severe menstrual pain than before, and many will also find that they have fewer or less dramatic side effects than with other hormonal contraceptive methods due to the low hormone dose. The most normal side effect, particularly with Kyleena, is spotting and irregular bleeding.

If you're worried that it will be painful to have the hormonal IUD inserted, it may be a good idea to take painkillers an hour before you're due to have it put in. Some will experience menstruation-like pains for a little while after insertion, but they quickly pass. After that, you won't notice it's there, except for the fact that you can feel two small strands of thread sticking out of your cervix in the deepest part of your vagina. This is what the doctor uses to remove the hormonal IUD when it's time to change it.

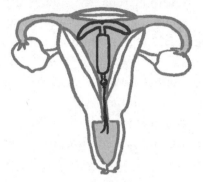

Estrogen-free contraceptive pills are a type of contraceptive pill that must be taken every day. You never take a break to have bleeding. Nor is there any need to take them at the same time every day. You are only at risk of pregnancy once it has been thirty-six hours since you took your last pill. The progestin in the estrogen-free hormonal pills works in the same way as in the contraceptive implant: it influences the pituitary gland in the brain to prevent ovulation. In addition, the mucus in the cervix becomes impenetrable and the uterine lining becomes thin.[7]

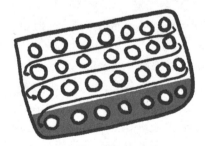

Mini pills are also a kind of pill you take every day without having a break for bleeding. The progestin dose in the mini pills is lower than in the estrogen-free contraceptive pills, so you have to be certain to take the pill at the same time every day. You have a window of about three hours, which makes it easier to use the pills incorrectly and risk pregnancy.[8] Some US brands of mini pills are: Orvette, Femulen, and Camila.

The *contraceptive injection* must be administered by a doctor or other health professional twelve weeks after the preceding dose. As such, you must visit a health professional for a new injection every third month. The hormonal injection contains a great deal of progestin, enough to prevent ovulation. It also works on the mucus in the cervix and on the uterine lining, which becomes thin. As a rule, the hormonal injection isn't recommended for women under the age of twenty-five, because the hormone dosage is so high that it affects the build-up of bone density in the body.[9]

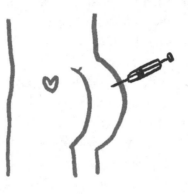

NON-HORMONAL CONTRACEPTION

Are you one of those people who wants a hormone-free alternative? The hormone-free methods have little in common with one another, and people have many reasons for choosing them. Some women choose this method because they have experienced side effects from hormonal contraception or they fear side effects and don't want to risk it. Protection against sexually transmitted diseases is a good reason to prefer condoms. Other women are concerned about hiding their contraceptive use from their partner or family and therefore prefer their menstrual cycle to continue as before.

CONDOMS

Condoms prevent the sperm cells from entering the uterus. The condom serves as a barrier and is therefore known as a barrier method. Today, the condom is the only easily available contraceptive method that can be used by men, though more male options are underway.

The condom is a kind of bag made of latex or similar material that is pulled onto the penis and collects the sperm when a man ejaculates. After sexual intercourse, it's important to hold the condom firmly in place when the penis is being withdrawn so that it doesn't end up left inside the vagina, sperm and all. Once that's done, it's just a matter of taking off the condom, tying a knot in it, and throwing it straight into the trash. Don't flush condoms down the toilet. They have a habit of floating back up again when you least expect it and that's no fun—either in shared accommodation or at your parents' house.

The condom is the only contraceptive method that protects you against sexually transmitted infections. In other words, condoms protect you against both disease and pregnancy. That makes it sound as if you should drop everything else and just use condoms all the time, but unfortunately many people have accidents when they use only condoms. The condom can split, slip off, or be destroyed. As a result, many people opt to combine condoms with other forms of contraception.

Many people also use condoms incorrectly, which means there's a greater chance of things going wrong. With this in mind, here's our recipe for perfect condom use.

CONDOM COURSE

1. Check the expiration date. An old condom is easier to break.
2. Open the condom package carefully. Be careful not to scratch the condom with sharp nails, teeth, or jewelry.
3. Once the penis is stiff, place the condom on top of it like a sombrero.
4. Squeeze the tip of the condom to push out the air. Trapped air may cause the condom to split. Carefully unroll the condom down over the penis.

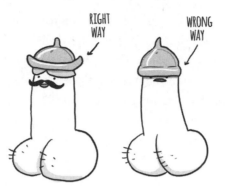

5. Hold the condom firmly in place when withdrawing the penis from the vagina, otherwise sperm may run out of it.
6. The condom should remain in use throughout intercourse to protect against pregnancy or sexually transmitted disease, and should only be used once.

There are other types of barrier methods that can be used by women. We've already introduced the diaphragm, i.e., the modern version of leaves and honey. There's also a kind of vaginal condom, which sits like a bag inside the vagina, instead of around the penis. This is called a female condom and also provides protection against disease. As far as we know, it isn't available on the market in Norway and is rarely used in our part of the world, but they are approved and available for purchase in the United States.[10]

FERTILITY AWARENESS–BASED METHODS—FIND YOUR FERTILE WINDOW

The period in which you can become pregnant during a menstrual cycle is called the fertile window. Some methods of contraception involve finding out when your fertile window is in order to avoid having sex when there's a chance of becoming pregnant.

There are different ways of doing this. You can use a menstrual calendar, measure your body temperature every morning, or examine your cervical mucus. People often combine these methods for greater reliability.

In recent years several applications have come on the market that help women keep track of their fertile windows and heighten the effectiveness of these methods. In Scandinavia we have Natural Cycles, which was recently approved by the EU as a contraceptive method. Other American apps that help users track their fertility by charting their menstrual cycles include Glow, Kindara, and Clue. Apps eliminate some of the possibility of miscalculation, and can use earlier temperature records to estimate the likelihood of pregnancy. A study financed by Natural Cycles found that their app increased effectiveness in typical use of the basal body temperature method from 75 percent to 92.5 percent, which means that 7.5 percent of users got pregnant in the course of a year. There are still very few studies on these apps with a representative group of participants, so we'll have to see if these numbers hold up in a more diverse group of users.

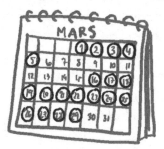

These methods are too unreliable to be recommended to women who absolutely do not want to become pregnant, because they require a lot from the user. According to the World Health Organization (WHO), 24 percent of women who use methods based on fertility awareness will become pregnant within a year with typical use—in other words, one in four.

Still, these methods may work well for women who accomplish the usage of these methods perfectly, as you can see in our table on the effectiveness of contraception (page 148). They are also great at making women more aware of how their bodies work and can be of significant help for women who are trying to become pregnant. They too can use the methods to identify their fertile window, making it easier to conceive.

People who calculate ovulation with a menstrual calendar use the information in the section on the menstrual cycle (pages 47–56) as their starting point. Ovulation generally happens at the same time every cycle, i.e., around fourteen days before menstruation.

The starting point for those who use the temperature method is that our body temperature changes slightly over the course of the menstrual cycle. By 0.6 degrees Fahrenheit to be precise! As you may recall, the menstrual cycle has two phases. One or two days before the second phase, your body temperature rises 0.6 degrees and remains elevated for around ten days. At the beginning of the second phase, large amounts of the LH hormone are released into the blood from the brain. The sharp increase in LH triggers ovulation, which generally occurs one or two days after the hormonal increase. In other words, ovulation occurs between two and four days after the body temperature rises. By measuring your temperature every day over a prolonged period you can find out when in your cycle you usually ovulate and use that as your basis for working out which days you are most fertile.

You can also tell from your cervical mucus when you are ovulating. For this to work you have to examine your discharge every day and look for changes. Just before ovulation your discharge becomes slick and slimy so that you can stretch it between your fingers, generally several centimeters. When ovulation has just occurred, your discharge will become white and creamy. This method requires you to be very familiar with your discharge, and to spend time studying how it alters over the course of your cycle. You should be aware that there are other reasons for changes in discharge apart from shifts in your cycle. For example various infections can affect the consistency, making it difficult to judge where you are in a cycle.[11]

Perhaps this sounds complicated—and indeed that's the problem. That is also why these methods aren't a great option for all women. We recommend types of contraception that are secure for everyone—methods with which you can't make mistakes.

Women who use fertility-based methods must live an extremely orderly life with plenty of time to examine mucus or take and record their temperature every morning, must have a will of steel when it comes to resisting sex at the wrong time (or must like using condoms), and must be prepared for the possibility of getting pregnant. If this sounds like you—and if you have an aversion to other birth control methods—go ahead and give fertility based–methods a try. But if you wish to avoid pregnancy at all costs, we advise you to choose something else.

If you already have problems with remembering pills, it is unrealistic to make fertility based–methods part of your daily routine. Even if the available apps make this aspect easier, there's a lot of measuring and recording involved. There's also leeway of several days, which allows a lot of opportunities to get it wrong. The method is less reliable in women without regular cycles. The menstrual cycle can be altered by external factors such as stress, weight changes, and illness. Young women often have more irregular cycles than older women, so the method will be even less suitable for young women, in addition to the fact that young women often live less organized lives.

COPPER IUD

A hormone-free alternative that we endorse is the copper IUD. Fewer than 1 percent of all women who use the copper IUD become pregnant in the course of a year. Like the hormonal IUD, the copper IUD is a little T-shaped object that is inserted in the uterus by a doctor or other health professional. The difference is that the copper IUD is coated in copper threads. The brand of copper IUD used in the United States is ParaGard and it can stay in your uterus for up to twelve years. It gives good protection against pregnancy the entire time. Two threads hang from the base of the copper IUD and stick out through the opening in the cervix so that you can check with your fingers whether the copper IUD is in place. The same goes for the hormonal IUD. The doctor uses these threads when the copper IUD is to be removed or replaced.

The initial cost for a copper IUD may be off-putting (the medical exam, the IUD, the insertion procedure, and follow-up visits to the doctor can range from $500 to $900 depending on health insurance coverage), but in comparison to birth control pills IUDs are less expensive over time.[12]

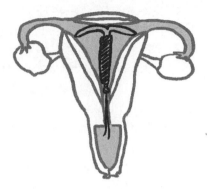

We don't know exactly why and how the copper IUD prevents pregnancy. What we do know is that the copper IUD causes a mild inflammation in the uterus, altering the environment to make it a hostile place for conception.[13] Somehow or other this prevents pregnancy. One theory is that the uterus begins to emit spermicidal substances as a result of the inflammation, or possibly that the copper itself kills the sperm.[14] Another theory is that the copper IUD prevents any fertilized eggs from attaching themselves to the uterine wall.

Women who use copper IUDs ovulate normally every month, unlike many of those who use hormonal contraception. The copper IUD doesn't have any effect on the brain or the ovaries. It only has a local effect in the uterus.

You won't get any hormonal side effects from a copper IUD, but that doesn't mean that it's free of side effects. Many women experience heavier bleeding and more severe menstrual pains than before. Two to ten out of one hundred women choose to remove the copper IUD in the first year as a result of these problems,[15] and the copper IUD is therefore not usually advisable for women who already suffer from such issues with their menstruation.

There are many myths about the copper IUD. The most widespread one is that you can't use it if you haven't previously given birth. It's perfectly fine to use both the hormonal IUD and the copper IUD even if you haven't had children, and you're welcome to try the copper IUD even if you're young. The copper IUD is an old and well-established form of contraception, and copper IUDs have become smaller and more reliable over the years.

From a purely practical standpoint it can be unpleasant having an IUD put in, since it has to be inserted through the narrow channel into the uterus. Many experience this as severe, short-term, menstruation-like pains. It may be worth taking painkillers in advance. Discuss this with your doctor before the insertion of the copper IUD.

If the threads at the bottom of the IUD suddenly disappear, you should contact your doctor. This may mean that the IUD has been pushed out of your uterus, resulting in your no longer being protected against pregnancy. Apparently, 5 to 10 percent of users find that the copper IUD falls out. In very rare cases the missing threads may indicate pregnancy. In the event of pregnancy the threads can in fact be drawn up into the uterus.

EMERGENCY CONTRACEPTION—PANIC STATIONS

Sunday morning. You had sex last night and you didn't use reliable contraception. You have no particular desire to get pregnant, and you're so scared your stomach aches. You're not the first person to experience this and you won't be the last either. Sometimes things go wrong, and that's why we have emergency contraception. This is something you can use after having had unprotected sex or if you've experienced contraceptive failure.

The definition of contraceptive failure varies depending on the type of contraception. It may be a missed pill, a vaginal ring that has fallen out, or a condom that has broken. It's important to become familiar with the method of contraception you're using so that you know when you've had contraceptive failure. How much time has to pass between two contraceptive pills before it's considered to be contraceptive failure? How long must the vaginal ring have been outside your vagina? Ask your doctor or nurse about the rules for contraceptive failure with your method of contraception.

Contraceptive failure when you're on hormonal contraception—for example a missed pill—often results in ovulation. Many people don't bother with emergency contraception after contraceptive failure because they don't understand that they risk getting pregnant. It may be several days since they had sex when they forget their pill. But remember that the sperm cell can survive five days inside the uterus while it's waiting for an egg. This means you can get pregnant from sex you had up to five days ago if you experience contraceptive failure that leads to an ovulation today.

In Norway people call emergency contraception the "regret pill." We should stop calling it that. "Regret pill" is a prim term that suggests pursed lips and raised eyebrows. It implies you've done something you should regret—but you really haven't. You've just had sex, and if it was a positive experience there's no reason to regret it. And, by the way, that feeling you get when you pick up the blister pack to take today's pill and discover you've missed three pills in the past week isn't regret: it's panic. That's why we've opted to call it the "panic pill" in this book.

We're not especially thrilled about the English term for it either—"the morning-after pill." It sounds nice and easy, as if you can take the pill every morning after sex instead of using contraception. But it's important not to resort to panic pills too easily. They're not as effective as regular contraception and there are a few side effects, although admittedly not dangerous ones. Emergency contraception should only be used when other contraception has failed. It shouldn't replace regular contraception.

In the United States, there are several brands of emergency contraceptive (EC) pills that may be available in your local pharmacy without showing ID. Regulations on the sale of EC have changed frequently, so it can be quite confusing.

Progestin-only EC (such as Plan B One-Step and its generic forms Take Action, Next Choice One Dose, and My Way) are approved for unrestricted sale on store shelves. Plan B One-Step usually costs about $50, and the generics cost about $40.

If you want to use your health insurance to purchase EC, the pharmacist at your local drugstore can help.

You can order a generic form of Plan B One-Step online at afterpill.com for $20 plus $5 shipping. This site does not offer expedited shipping, so it's not meant for emergency use. Buy it to keep it on hand for future use.

Ella is sold by prescription only, regardless of age. You can also order ella online at KwikMed or prjktruby.com for $67, including next-day shipping.[16]

PANIC PILL TYPE I: LEVONORGESTREL

The first type of panic pill contains a substance called levonorgestrel, which is a kind of progestin. In other words it contains the same substance as hormonal contraception, only the progestin dose is much higher. This is the most common type of emergency contraception. In the United States, it's called Plan B One-Step and sells for about $50. Generic versions include Take Action and Next Choice One Dose, and are priced at about $40.

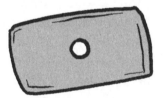

Panic pill type I works by postponing ovulation. The problem is that it doesn't work if you've already ovulated, or if you're just about to ovulate. As you may remember from the chapter about the menstrual cycle, women experience a dramatic increase in the hormone LH just before ovulation. Once the rise in LH is already underway, pills containing levonorgestrel won't be able to stop ovulation.

As we have discussed previously, it's difficult to know whether you've ovulated or not. Only women with totally regular cycles know more or less when they ovulate, but many factors can disturb a regular menstrual cycle.

So this pill isn't entirely reliable, although it does reduce the chance that you'll get pregnant, so it's definitely sensible to take it. The sooner you take the pill the better. It's best to take it within twenty-four hours. That said, the panic pill can be effective for up to three days (seventy-two hours) after unprotected sex or contraceptive failure. The chances of the pill being effective decrease as more time passes so it's a good idea to keep one in your toiletry bag at all times. It's perfectly fine to take a pill containing levonorgestrel several times in the course of a single menstrual cycle.[17]

Advantage: availability, doesn't affect other contraception, may be taken several times in a cycle
Disadvantage: less reliable
Remember: pregnancy test after three weeks!

PANIC PILL TYPE II: ULIPRISTAL ACETATE

The second type of panic pill contains a substance called ulipristal acetate. This substance influences the way natural progesterone functions in the body. In the United States, pills containing ulipristal acetate are known as "ella." This pill is effective for up to five days (120 hours) after unprotected sex or contraceptive failure. In the US, ella is prescription only, but most women can obtain it easily from a women's health clinic.[18]

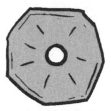

Like panic pills containing levonorgestrel, ulipristal acetate pills postpone ovulation. The difference between the two types of panic pill is that this variant can be taken much closer to ovulation and still be effective. You can take it right up until ovulation. In other words, pills with ulipristal acetate work effectively even if the rise in LH is already underway in your body. This makes the pill more effective and it will prevent more pregnancies. However, this pill will not be effective either if you've already ovulated.

Of course, there is one major disadvantage with this pill, too. The main problem is that it reacts badly with hormonal contraception. First and foremost, it affects the way your regular contraception works after you've taken it. This means you have to use condoms for a while after taking the panic pill, because there's a chance that your hormonal contraception won't work properly. How long you have to do that for will depend on what kind of contraception you use.

Likewise, the kind of hormonal contraception you use can influence how effective the emergency contraception pill is. This means that you shouldn't use hormonal contraception after taking ella. In fact, new research shows that use of hormonal contraception can disrupt the panic pill's effect on ovulation, preventing it from being postponed after all. You should wait until five days after taking ella before starting or continuing to use hormonal contraception.[19]

Emergency contraception using ulipristal acetate should only be used once in any menstrual cycle, because no research has been done into the use of several pills in a single cycle. This doesn't mean the pill is dangerous, just that nobody knows whether it's effective more than once a cycle. Since the pill influences other hormonal contraception, it can also affect the use of panic pill type I with levonorgestrel if you try to take it right after using ulipristal acetate. If you've already taken ulipristal acetate, it's best to use the copper IUD if you experience another failure.[20]

Advantage: better and longer effect than the levonorgestrel pill
Disadvantage: reacts badly with hormonal contraception
Remember: pregnancy test after three weeks!

COPPER IUD

Although the copper IUD is the safest form of emergency contraception, and it is said to be 99 percent effective for this purpose, it's rarely used. In other countries, including Norway, we encourage usage of the copper IUD as emergency contraception, but in the US the high price may make it an inconvenient option for many women. The copper IUD works by preventing fertilized eggs from attaching themselves to the uterus.

The copper IUD is inserted into the uterus by health professionals, so after you've had unprotected sex you can request an emergency appointment with your doctor and explain what's happened. You can also go to an urgent care center or a women's clinic. The copper IUD is effective for five days (120 hours) after unprotected sex or contraceptive failure. It works because the fertilized egg doesn't attach itself to the wall of the uterus before the sixth day after ovulation, so in some cases it's possible to use the copper IUD as emergency contraception more than five days after intercourse, if you know when ovulation occurred. The copper IUD must be used at latest on the fifth day after ovulation.

The good thing about the copper IUD, apart from the fact that it's extremely effective as emergency contraception, is that you can then leave it in your uterus and use it as regular contraception. If you don't want it as your regular method of contraception, it's also possible to have it removed after a short time.[21]

Advantage: highly reliable, can serve as contraception for the next twelve years
Disadvantage: availability, requires a prescription, and must be inserted by a doctor

WHAT TO REMEMBER

Many people think they're perfectly safe after taking the panic pill, but that isn't true!

Emergency contraception reduces the risk of getting pregnant, but it doesn't work nearly as well as regular contraception. It's important to take a pregnancy test after using emergency contraception. We recommend that you take the test whether you have menstrual bleeding or not. If your partner or a female friend is the one who's taken the panic pill, it's helpful to remind her to take a test.

For the pregnancy test to be reliable you have to wait at least three weeks after using emergency contraception before taking it. There's no point taking a test immediately after using emergency contraception, because it's impossible to detect whether you've become pregnant or not so soon afterward.

Emergency contraception has side effects. The most common one is irregular bleeding. Panic pills postpone ovulation, which also delays your period. It isn't dangerous to have irregular bleeding, but it can be a nuisance. Luckily it's not a long-term problem and will pass. Some people also find that panic pills make them nauseated. If you vomit shortly after taking the pill, you'll have to take another one. Follow the instructions on the patient information leaflet and from your doctor.

The copper IUD doesn't contain hormones, but even so it's pretty common to have changes in your regular bleeding pattern at the beginning. If you intend to keep the copper IUD as your regular contraception and you experience bleeding changes, we recommend that you wait to see how things are after three months. The bleeding often stabilizes over time.

ARE SOME METHODS OF CONTRACEPTION BETTER THAN OTHERS?

We talk a lot about how different we are and how different methods of contraception are good for different women, but that doesn't mean that all types of contraception are equally good at preventing pregnancy. There's a reason why leaves and honey in the vagina have gone out of fashion, and fertility awareness–based methods are responsible for many unwanted pregnancies. That's just the way it is.

Women who use the contraceptive implant have the lowest risk of becoming pregnant, closely followed by the hormonal IUD. In other words, these two types of contraception are the best. A lot of people wonder how this quality is measured. How do we determine how good the different types of contraception are? And what does it actually mean to say that the implant is better than the pill? To clarify: When we say "best" we mean how effective the method of contraception is, i.e., how good it is at preventing pregnancy. We're not talking about side effects or how many people like the method of contraception. Whether or not you like the method is personal. But how well it prevents pregnancy can be measured objectively, simply by seeing how many women have become pregnant while they've been using the particular method of contraception in a study. It's far from certain that you'll prefer the contraceptive method that is objectively the best. The aim is to find a method of contraception that is as reliable as possible and that you are also happy with.

Researchers use something called the Pearl Index when they're assessing and comparing different methods of contraception. The Pearl Index is the number of women in a group of one hundred users of contraception who become pregnant in the course of a year.*

If for example you want to investigate the effectiveness of a new kind of contraceptive pill, you ask a group of women to test the pill and then see how many of them do and don't become pregnant while they're using it. By using results from many such studies, statisticians can rank the methods of contraception according to how effective they are. But what causes the difference in effectiveness between the different methods of contraception?

Two factors contribute to how well a method of contraception works. The first factor relates to how it is used. Because it's possible to use some of the methods of contraception incorrectly, that makes them less effective than those that cannot be used incorrectly. We call this factor "user error."

Take the withdrawal method, for example. The aim is for a man to withdraw from a woman's vagina right before he comes, so that his sperm ends up anywhere but there. But as many of us have found out, it's only too easy to pull out *after* rather than *before* coming.

---

* There's a common misconception that the theoretically highest index is one hundred, as if it were a matter of percentages. But if all the women in a study became pregnant in the course of their first cycle, the Pearl Index would actually be around 1,200. It's pretty confusing and actually not especially important unless you're a total nerd. Like us.

In the heat of the moment it's so tempting to carry on just a *little* longer, but if you mess up one time, that can be enough to get pregnant. The possibility of using the withdrawal method incorrectly makes it difficult to rely on, and it is far from popular among health professionals and users who absolutely don't want to get pregnant. Human capacity for error always comes into play even though perfect use would have been entirely effective.

The contraceptive pill, one of the most common methods of contraception, is also an offender when it comes to user error. In fact, user error is its middle name. It's incredibly easy to miss a pill or two. Every woman who's ever woken up in another person's bed far away from her toothbrush and pack of pills knows that. Many women who get pregnant when they're using contraceptive pills do so because of the pill-free week. They get out of the routine of taking a pill every day and then they mess up on how long the break should be. Missing a pill can happen to anybody. All of us can have an absentminded day, and some people are absentminded every day.

The contraceptive implant, on the other hand, is more effective because it sits in your arm and does its job without you having to do anything at all. It's impossible to forget the implant other than when you have to change it, and that's only once every three years. So there's no user error with the implant. It works perfectly, regardless of your routines and your memory.

Some people may think it's unfair to say that methods of contraception are bad just because the users mess up; after all, that isn't the method's fault, is it? You may well think that, but we take the view that there's no point respecting the nonexistent feelings of methods of contraception. Studies show that humans often end up doing things wrong whenever there's any possibility for it, and this has an impact on the effectiveness of the method of contraception.

The second factor that determines effectiveness is the actual quality of the method. Many people think that sterilization is the most effective thing you can do if you don't want to have (more) children. When a woman is sterilized, her fallopian tubes are cut so that the egg cannot pass from the ovary to the uterus, but even after sterilization one in two hundred women actually become pregnant in the following year. Both the contraceptive implant and the hormonal IUD are more effective than that. This type of error, which has to do with the means of contraception itself and not the person using it, is called "method error."

Pretty much nobody gets pregnant using the implant, but nothing is black and white in medicine. Someone somewhere will become pregnant regardless of which method she's using. Unfortunately, you can never say never as long as you're a woman who has sex with a man; but you can say "almost never" and that'll just have to do.

Since there are two different kinds of error connected to methods of contraception, user error and method error, their effectiveness is also measured in two different ways. We distinguish between "perfect use" and "actual use" of a method of contraception. Perfect use means that the person using the method of contraception has used it in a completely error-free way. There is no user error, no missed pill, no late withdrawal, and no vaginal ring falling in the toilet during a boozy night out on the town. On the other hand, actual use is the result when women do their best to use contraceptive methods correctly, but still end up making a mistake here and there.

The difference between perfect and actual use can be anywhere between major and nonexistent, depending on how many mistakes it's possible to make with that particular method.

If your life has a good routine, if you're not the least bit scatter-brained or absentminded, and if you have steely control over, for example, contraceptive pills, it may be that your risk of pregnancy lies closer to the Pearl Index for "perfect use" than "actual use." You're the only one who knows yourself well enough to know that. But if you have a slightly more unpredictable lifestyle, it may be worth considering a method of contraception that works regardless of how many mistakes you make. Methods of contraception without user error, for example the implant and the copper IUD/hormonal IUD, are equally effective when it comes to perfect and actual use because actual use is perfect without you having to make any effort at all.

So which methods of contraception are best? Below you'll find a table with a selection of the different methods. The figures are provided by the WHO. These were updated in 2016 but may change as researchers find new methods of contraception or carry out new research into existing methods.

It may be helpful to know how good the different methods of contraception perform in tests when you're making your choice. However, we advise as many women as possible to try the most effective methods: the ones that have a long-acting effect and no possibility of user error.

Effectiveness of Methods of Contraception[22, 23, 24]

	PERFECT USE How many become pregnant	TYPICAL USE How many become pregnant	Effectiveness of method of contraception
Contraceptive implant	0.05%	0.05%	99.95%
Hormonal IUD	0.2%	0.2%	99.8%
Sterilization, men	0.1%	0.1%	99.9%
Sterilization, women	0.5%	0.5%	99.5%
Copper IUD	0.6%	0.8%	99.2–99.4%
Contraceptive injection	0.3%	3%	97–99.7%
Contraceptive pill	0.3%	8%	92–99.7%
Condom	2%	15%	85–98%
Withdrawal	4%	27%	73–96%
Fertility awareness–based methods	No perfect use data available as the methods differ.	24%	76%
Menstruation calendar	5%	12%	88–95%
Basal body temperature method	1%	25%	75–99%
Cervical secretion monitoring method	4%	14%	86–96%
No protection		85–90%	10–15%

PERIODS ON HORMONAL CONTRACEPTION

Hormonal contraception affects your menstrual cycle. You'll notice it because your monthly bleeding will alter. Most women get lighter or shorter bleeding, but that's not true for everybody. Bleeding may also become irregular or disappear entirely. A lot of women find this part spooky because there are a lot of myths about ceasing or skipping periods. *Doesn't the bleeding come because it's natural?*, many people think. *Don't our bodies need it? Should we really be messing with Mother Nature in this way?*

As you may remember from the chapter on periods (page 43) there's nothing to suggest that menstrual bleeding in itself constitutes an advantage for you. That's certainly true if you're using hormonal contraception. Most types of hormonal contraception will actually stop the menstrual cycle entirely, by pressing the pause button in your pituitary gland. So the bleeding that happens is no longer normal menstruation, either, but what we call withdrawal bleeding.

Let's start with what happens with your period if you use combined pills. The researchers who designed contraceptive pills almost sixty years ago built in one pill-free week every month precisely so that women could have withdrawal bleeding. They thought it would be easier to accept the pill as a method of contraception if the hormones produced something resembling a normal menstrual cycle, with regular bleeding every fourth week. But even though the contraception imitates a natural cycle, it isn't "natural." Nor is the bleeding natural, and there's nothing unnatural about skipping it.

Usually it's estrogen that causes the endometrium to grow and this mucous membrane is what later becomes your period. The estrogen in the combined products makes the endometrium grow a little bit each month, so most women who use combined contraceptives will have withdrawal bleeding when they take a break of seven days or fewer from hormonal pills, the contraceptive patch, or the vaginal ring, even if they don't have a normal cycle. Endometrial growth is less than normal and that's why it isn't necessary to bleed as often as when you're not using contraception. Once a month may be superfluous for many women.

If you're using combined products, you can skip menstruation as many times as you like or even use the pills continuously and have the bleeding whenever you feel like it. The progestin in the combined products binds the endometrium so that it doesn't bleed out.

If you're using combined products and skip the withdrawal bleeding often enough, you'll probably eventually get what's called breakthrough bleeding. The progestin binds the endometrium for as long as it can, but in the end it becomes too much. Breakthrough bleeding means that you bleed while you're on hormones—in other words outside the short hormone break you can take when you're using the pill, the vaginal ring, or the contraceptive patch. This can involve either spotting, i.e., irregular light bleeding—generally just spots on your underwear—or heavier menstruation-like bleeding. This is normal and all it means is that it's time to take a break for a maximum of seven days; then you can go back to skipping the withdrawal bleeding again.

Many women think the monthly bleeding you get when using hormonal methods can show whether you're pregnant or not and that if you skip it for too long, this may conceal a potential pregnancy, but that's not correct. In fact, it's possible to stop bleeding entirely when using combined products even if you do take a pill-free week in between. This doesn't have anything to do with whether or not you're pregnant. What's more, it's possible to have light bleeding during a pregnancy. Bleeding on hormonal contraception is often light and not the same as a regular period. So you could be pregnant even if you bleed lightly in the pill-free week. The central message is that you should trust the method of contraception you're using. Combined contraceptives are effective if used correctly, but if anything changes and you suspect pregnancy the only way to check is by taking a pregnancy test.

A lot of women suffer from frequent breakthrough bleeding, and this can be a nuisance over the long term. Some may find it helps to change their contraceptive method. If you're on the Pill, it could help to change from a variant with a low dose of estrogen to types that have a slightly higher dose. The pills with the highest estrogen dose are best at controlling bleeding. For example, many women will experience less bleeding on higher estrogen doses (Ortho-Novum, Triphasil, or Ortho Tri-Cyclen in the US) than on Loestrin. You can discuss with a doctor which type you should switch to.

Periods on progestin contraception are very different from periods on combined contraceptives. The main difference is that you can't decide what your cycle will be like, and you can't change or control it along the way. This is because you take the same dose of hormone every day, without taking a break. If you do take a break, you lose your protection. This means that you'll have bleeding when the progestin can no longer bind the endometrium, and that can happen at any time. All bleeding when you are on progestin contraception is, in practice, breakthrough bleeding since there's no time set aside to have withdrawal bleeding.

Progestin will bind the uterine lining, making it more difficult for it to bleed out. At the same time the mucous membrane becomes thinner than usual. Since there's no estrogen in progestin contraception there's nothing to tell the uterine lining that it should grow. As a result there's no certainty you'll have any bleeding at all, although many women do. After all, estrogen occurs naturally in the body, too.

When you start using a progestin contraceptive it's a bit like playing Russian roulette with your menstrual cycle. You don't know in advance what it will be like, but it will be one of three alternatives: regular bleeding, no bleeding, or irregular bleeding.

A lot of people think all women who use the implant or the hormonal IUD stop menstruating altogether, and many choose this method of contraception for precisely that reason. Although a lot of women end up without bleeding, there's also a possibility you'll end up with extremely irregular bleeding or a totally regular cycle. Whatever happens, the amount of bleeding will be less than it was without hormonal contraception.

As with the combined products, the fact of bleeding while you're on progestin contraceptive doesn't rule out pregnancy. We've had questions from young women who religiously take a pregnancy test every third month because they've stopped having periods as a result of contraception. This is unnecessary and expensive. Bleeding (or the lack of it) is not a good indicator of pregnancy when you're using progestin contraceptives. Take a pregnancy test if you've experienced contraceptive failure or are uncertain whether you're protected against pregnancy, but otherwise, there's no need to.

Although the copper IUD isn't a hormonal method, you may have side effects related to your period. Unlike with hormonal contraception, which leads to lighter bleeding, many will find they have heavier bleeding and more severe menstrual pains when they use the copper IUD. This is particularly true for women who have previously suffered from heavy, prolonged, or painful bleeding. As many as one in ten women opt to remove the copper IUD in the first year as a result of these problems.[25]

HOW DO I SKIP MY PERIOD?

Sometimes it's not convenient to have a period. That could be because you're going on a beach vacation, a camping trip, or because you can't deal with the blood and pains in the last week before your exam. These are things all women who menstruate can relate to, particularly those who suffer heavier bleeding and a lot of pain. When it's not convenient you can try to postpone the bleeding.

It's always easiest to postpone bleeding if you use combined contraceptives—in other words combined pills, the contraceptive patch, or the vaginal ring.[26] Others may use prescribed medication that's designed to postpone your period.[27]

HERE'S WHAT TO DO

Monophasic-type combined pills: Normally you'll take your hormone-containing pills for twenty-one or twenty-four days before taking a hormone-free break of either seven or four days, depending on which type of monophasic pill you're taking. During these pill-free days you'll have bleeding. If you want to skip the bleeding, you can go straight to a new pack once you've finished up all the hormone-containing pills in your current one. So if you're using a pack that contains twenty-one hormone pills (for example Ortho-Novum or Loestrin), you won't have the usual pill-free week. If sugar pills are included, making a total of twenty-eight pills in the pack, you can throw them away. If you use Yaz or Zoely, which operate with twenty-four hormone pills and a four-day break, you can skip the break and go directly to a new pack of twenty-four hormone pills. If you're taking multiphasic pills such as Seasonale you can also skip your period, but in this case you'll need a slightly more thorough explanation. We encourage those of you using these pills to visit a doctor or nurse if you have questions and to check the patient information leaflet for instructions.

Vaginal ring: Normally you keep a vaginal ring in for three weeks before taking a one-week break, which we can call a ring-free or hormone-free week. During this week you'll have bleeding. If you want to skip it, you can insert a new ring into your vagina after three weeks without having a ring-free week.

Contraceptive patch: The contraceptive patch is normally changed once a week for three weeks before having a patch-free week in the fourth week. During this week you'll have bleeding. To skip the bleeding, put a new patch on in the fourth week instead of having a patch-free week.

WHAT'S THE BEST WAY TO USE CONTRACEPTIVE PILLS?

The contraceptive pill can be a lot of trouble, but it's still a popular method. As mentioned earlier, it's possible to become pregnant while you're using contraceptive pills, mainly because it's so easy to use them incorrectly.

What's cool is that there's a way of using contraceptive pills that involves less risk of pregnancy, fewer bleeding abnormalities, and lighter bleeding. This method works for all combined products, including the contraceptive patch and the contraceptive implant. People using multiphasic pills must follow separate instructions from a doctor or nurse.

Contraceptive pills and other combined products are effective as long as you use them correctly. As you know, combined contraceptives are designed with a built-in break. You use the hormones for three weeks (twenty-one days), followed by one week (seven days) without hormones, either without any pills at all or taking sugar pills. During the seven days you'll have withdrawal bleeding. If you're using Yaz or Zoely, you'll take hormone pills for twenty-four days and have a four-day break.

Twenty-one and seven or twenty-four and four are immensely important numbers when it comes to combined contraception, because they mark two important limits.

When you use combined contraception, you must take hormones for *at least twenty-one or twenty-four days* in order for the contraceptive to be effective. If you use hormones for fewer than twenty-one or twenty-four days in a row—for example if you forget the last two pills in the pack and end up with nineteen or twenty-two days instead of twenty-one or twenty-four—there's a danger that you'll lose your protection and ovulate. Then you could get pregnant. Twenty-one or twenty-four days of hormones therefore means you must take them for *at least* twenty-one or twenty-four days. There's no problem with using hormones for longer. As long as you're over the limit, you can take the pills for thirty, fifty, or one hundred days in a row. It's entirely up to you.

The number seven (or four if you're using Zoely or Yaz) is a limit that means that the break can *be a maximum of seven or four days*. It must not be any longer. If you take a longer break than this from the hormones, you will not be protected against pregnancy. There's no problem with taking a break of, say, three days. If, for example, you have short bleeding, for only two days, you can start on hormones again after just a two-day break. But you must never take a break longer than seven or four days. If you do, you may ovulate and then you're in danger of getting pregnant.

Since so many unplanned pregnancies result from messing up on the pill-free week, it can only be a good thing to reduce the number of pill-free weeks. This will make the contraception more effective.

You'll probably have breakthrough bleeding once you've been skipping your period for several months. You can solve this by using combined pills continuously and taking breaks when you need to. That way, you can formulate a cycle that suits you, with as few periods of bleeding as possible.

Take hormones continuously until you have bleeding and then take a break to get the bleeding over with. That break may well be shorter than seven or four days. After the break, start taking hormones again and use them right up until you have new breakthrough bleeding. This is absolutely fine as long as you never take fewer than twenty-one or twenty-four pills in a row. If you have bleeding after, say, ten days of hormone pills, you have to continue until you've taken twenty-one or twenty-four in order to be protected against pregnancy.

HORMONAL CONTRACEPTION—BUT ISN'T IT DANGEROUS?

You've probably noticed that "natural" is the new ideal. Words like *detox, parabens, juicing,* and *superfood* have become commonplace. The message of the self-proclaimed health gurus is clear: "Artificial" additives are no good for your body. You shouldn't mess with them.

Overnight, green juice has become the hottest fashion accessory and, at the same time, hormonal contraception has gone out of vogue. Young women have become afraid of using contraceptive pills because they're worried about sinister side effects. More and more, we hear people saying they have hormonal contraception intolerance, as if it was an allergy. Others ask whether it's healthy to take a hormone break, a detox, to flush the "unnatural substances" out of their body.

At a time when there's a growing focus on the pure and the natural, lots of people feel doctors aren't taking their concerns about

side effects seriously—the medical profession trivializes their problems or tries to sweep them under the rug. The result is that many
women have a nagging uncertainty about how safe their method of
contraception actually is, and end up seeking out information from
unreliable sources.

Around one third of all women stop taking the Pill in the first six
months after they started.[28] Of these, around half do so as a result
of what they experience as side effects.[29] It can be frightening to feel
that your body is changing if you don't understand why it's happening or what it means. Since knowledge breeds confidence, we think
you should have sufficient information about both the positive and
negative sides of hormonal contraception in order to make good
choices for your body.

At the same time, it's important for us to add some nuance to
the scary images that have emerged recently. Sometimes the media
gives the impression that we don't know about the side effects
linked to hormonal contraception, as if we were playing Russian
roulette with the health of young women. Fortunately, this is incorrect and sensational. You can be confident that the pack of pills you
pick up at the pharmacy contains one of the most carefully studied
medications in the world. Researchers have huge amounts of statistical material to examine since many millions of women have taken
birth control pills over vast swathes of the planet since the 1960s.
Unknown, serious, long-term effects from hormonal contraception
would have been discovered long ago if they existed, particularly
when you consider that the first pills that came on the market contained up to five times as much hormone as the ones we have today.

WHAT IS A SIDE EFFECT?

Before we start to talk about individual side effects, you need to
understand what a side effect is. A medication is designed to have
a particular effect on the body and that's why we take it. In the case
of hormonal contraception, the reason we take it is that we wish to
prevent pregnancy. Side effects are all the other effects the medication has on the body, which can be both positive and negative. For

example, many women find that they have a lot fewer breakouts when they use hormonal contraception, which is a side effect that is perceived as positive. Blood clots, on the other hand, are a side effect nobody wants to have.

In the film *Sliding Doors* (1998) we follow Gwyneth Paltrow's two parallel destinies: in one scenario she catches her train to work one morning, and in the other she misses it. This little detail has major consequences for the way her life turns out. Our body works the same way. It's so complicated and complex that it's impossible to affect a single function without creating ripple effects in other parts of the body at the same time. The mere presence of side effects doesn't mean that a medication is harmful. It means that it's working. If anybody ever claims that a medicine or treatment has no side effects, they're either lying or the substance has no effect whatsoever.

Doctors and health authorities are very concerned about side effects. We know they are a necessary evil, but the aim is to keep them at as low a level as possible. This is why it's extremely difficult to get medications approved for use. The drug manufacturer must first prove that the positive effects of the medicine will have the greatest possible likelihood of outweighing the negative effects. Years of studies and controlled experiments lie behind any new medication, precisely because we must know for sure what side effects you can expect when you take it.

In Norway, after a medication becomes available for use, it's carefully monitored by the Norwegian Medicines Agency, which is independent of the pharmaceutical industry, so that any unknown side effects can be detected early on. If patients experience a side effect, they and their doctor can report it to the agency. If there's any suspicion of a serious side effect having been overlooked—for example that use of the pill over many years causes cancer—new studies are launched. The same thing happens in the United States. The US Food and Drug Administration approves and carefully monitors all prescription medications in America. All serious side effects should be reported to your physician or ER. If appropriate, the medical professional will file a report with the FDA.

THE NOCEBO EFFECT

Why don't people automatically believe it when a lot of women report the same side effect from a medication? Why wouldn't the health care establishment trust women when they say they've experienced a side effect? One of the reasons health professionals insist on further investigation is something called a nocebo effect.

Most people have heard of placebos—i.e., situations in which people experience real, positive effects from something that doesn't actually work just because they expect that it will. For example, there's a reason why many medicines come in brightly colored capsules: It has been found people experience greater effects if the pills they take look sophisticated! This is also one of the reasons why doctors wear white coats and generally keep their stethoscope in sight around their neck. The coat and the stethoscope create associations of healing and professional competence in the patient. This alone can contribute to improving patients' health.

The nocebo effect, from the Latin for "I will harm," works the opposite way. Here a sugar pill causes physical problems because you believe it contains active substances. In fact, around a quarter of all patients experience negative side effects when they receive placebo treatment, in other words no treatment at all.[30] The same thing happens if a doctor tells a patient that a medication may have a particular negative effect. More people report this effect than usual without it actually being caused by the medicine. It can often be as simple as people attributing normal symptoms to the medicine. One study by Reidenberg and Lowenthal found that only 19 percent of healthy people who weren't taking any medicines had been entirely problem-free for the previous three days. Thirty-nine percent, however, had experienced fatigue, 14 percent had had a headache, and 5 percent had felt dizzy.

A study from Yale University found that highly educated women overestimated the dangers of hormonal contraception. At the same time they were unaware of all the positive health benefits it offers—for example, reduced risk of ovarian and endometrial cancer.[31] These negative expectations can become a self-fulfilling prophecy.

With this in mind it may be easier to understand why doctors are skeptical when a lot of women suddenly report a new side effect from an established medication such as the Pill. They know that it may simply be the result of too much negative publicity.[32] More research is the only way to find out whether what's being reported is a real side effect that has not been discovered before or just a nocebo effect.

EVERYTHING HAS A RISK

Begin by taking out the patient information leaflet for your hormonal contraception. There you'll find a long list of side effects, arranged according to how common they are. The most common apparently affect between one in ten and one in one hundred users. These include things like headaches, mood swings, and breast tenderness. The side effects that affect between one in one hundred and one in one thousand are listed next. The farther down the list you get, the more disturbing the reading.

The first thing to be aware of when you read this list is who wrote the patient information leaflet: the manufacturer of the medication. You might think that perhaps they're trying to hide side effects from you, but the opposite is true. Drug manufacturers lay it on thick when it comes to possible side effects so that they can't be taken to court by dissatisfied customers. Some of the effects included in the patient information leaflet are things that have been reported by women using the medication but haven't necessarily been proven to have been caused by the drug. We'll come back to this later. Others are side effects that we know are caused by hormonal contraception.

The other thing you must be clear about is an understanding of the word *risk*. When we hear the word *risk*, it's easy to think that something dangerous will happen, but it's actually just a warning of the *chance* of something happening.

To grasp the concept of risk, a short course in statistics is warranted. When we talk about side effects, what is known as the relative risk often hogs all the attention. Relative risk is how much the chance of having a side effect increases when you take a medication compared with when you don't take it. For example, you may read about the danger of blood clots being between two and four times higher for contraceptive pill users than for those who don't use them. This sounds dramatic. Just imagine the tabloid headline: "Life-Threatening Pill! Four Times the Likelihood of Blood Clots!" But it's actually not dramatic at all.

The fact that's most interesting for us as individuals is something called the "absolute risk." But the tabloids aren't as interested in this figure, because it would often result in boring headlines: "Minimal Chance of Blood Clots from the Pill! Meet the Girl Who Was Incredibly Unlucky and Got One Anyway." Absolute risk is the actual likelihood that there will be a side effect when you use, say, the contraceptive pill, without any comparison with people who aren't taking it. This presents a much more understandable and realistic picture of the danger you're exposed to.

What's the likelihood that you'll have a blood clot when you're taking the contraceptive pill? Although the relative risk indicates that users of the pill are at between two and four times *higher risk* of developing blood clots than those who don't use it, the likelihood that you'll actually develop a blood clot, the absolute risk, is somewhere between 0.0005 percent and 0.001 percent per year. This means that between 50 to 100 in 100,000 women on the contraceptive pill will develop a blood clot every year. In other words, even if you take the Pill you'd have to be incredibly unlucky to develop a blood clot.

NORMAL SIDE EFFECTS OF HORMONAL CONTRACEPTION

Now that we have a little bit of background information about side effects, we can start to deal with hormonal contraception in particular. Let's begin with the most common things first: the side effects that affect between 1 and 10 percent, such as headaches, dizziness, and breast tenderness. These are not dangerous side effects, but they can still be unpleasant. Nobody gets all these side effects, and many women don't experience any of them. The fact that one to ten people have these side effects means that ninety to ninety-nine people don't.

It's also important to be aware that there's no connection between the common and the dangerous side effects. If you suffer a common side effect, you are not at higher risk for the dangerous ones.

The common side effects tend to pass after several months' use, so we recommend trying a new method of contraception for three months before giving up and trying another one. If you still find you're having problems with the side effects after a three-month period, you should try another brand or another form of contraception.

The fact is that people react differently to different brands and methods. A product that gave your friend a pounding headache may be perfect for you. You'll only find out if you try it for yourself. As we explained earlier, there are different subtypes of progestin in the different products and they act on us slightly differently. There's also a difference between using a method of contraception that contains only progestin, such as the hormonal IUD and the implant, or a combined product that also contains estrogen. Even if you had many side effects with one product, this doesn't mean that you're "intolerant" of hormonal contraception in general. There's a high likelihood that there are other kinds that won't cause you problems. You simply have to ensure that you choose a method with a different variant of progestin; your doctor can help you with this.

Contraceptives that contain estrogen have particular side effects that are quite common.[33,34] In fact, these are very reminiscent of the things you can experience when you're pregnant! First on the list are nausea and dizziness. As with pregnant women, these symptoms pass pretty quickly, but if you're very bothered by them at the start it might make sense to take the pills at mealtimes or before going to bed.

Estrogen can also lead to increased discharge. It should not look or smell any different from normal; there's just more of it. A few people also get leg cramps. We don't know why that happens, but we do know it isn't dangerous. One less common side effect is that small amounts of milk may seep out of your nipples.

Another side effect of estrogen-based contraception is pigmentation. Although this is a side effect women experience on estrogen contraception, it's probably mostly caused by the progestin in the contraceptive. Pigmentation, technically known as *melasma*, manifests itself in darker brown patches on the skin. These occur when sunbathing, either outdoors or in a tanning booth. It's normal to get this kind of pigmentation during pregnancy, when it's also caused by natural hormones. If you have this problem, wearing a high-factor sunscreen can help.[35] Another alternative is to try a contraceptive containing a different progestin.

Estrogen also has positive effects. You may have heard people say that pregnant women glow. Clearer skin is actually one effect of estrogen. If you have problems with acne, combined products can help. Contraceptives containing only progestin can, however, have the opposite effect, causing greasy skin, greasy hair, and acne in some women. This is a factor that may be important for some people when choosing a method of contraception.

Contraception containing estrogen is, in fact, often used as part of the treatment for girls with polycystic ovary syndrome, a common condition that we'll come back to in a later chapter (pages 208–12).

Another positive side effect of contraceptives containing estrogen is that they give you the option to take control of your period. This means you get fewer cramps, spend less money on tampons, and often experience less severe PMS.

There's a myth that hormonal contraception causes you to put on weight. One reason for this myth is that many women start using contraception during a phase of life in which the body is undergoing dramatic change: puberty. Another reason may be that a lot of women put on weight when they get into a relationship. They think these extra partner pounds are due to their contraception, forgetting that suddenly they're spending a lot more time on the sofa cuddling, with a bag of chips on their lap and five seasons of *Game of Thrones* on the TV. You don't actually gain weight from hormonal contraception,[36] but it's all too easy to lay the blame there.

Another common early side effect is *edema*, which is the medical term for swelling. Simply put, this means that water accumulates in your body. Both estrogen and progestin may be to blame, so all hormonal products can have this effect, not just the combined products. Fluid retention is one of the reasons why some women think they're putting on weight when they start using hormonal contraception, but you haven't gained fat, you just have extra water in your body.

Your breasts may also retain fluid, becoming larger and more sensitive. Another unexpected side effect is that contact lens users may find their lenses suddenly don't fit right. This is because a little extra water is retained in the eye as well, and so the cornea, on which the contact lens lies, changes shape. The increased amount of water in the body may also lead to headaches.

Many women who use the Pill, patch, or ring only have headaches during the week of bleeding, in other words the week when they stop taking hormonal contraception.[37] This is very common and it's a bit like the headache you get when you haven't had your regular morning cup of coffee. The headache is a sign that you're missing something you're used to getting, in this case hormones. To reduce these pains you can simply skip or shorten the hormone-free interval to a few days. As mentioned earlier, there's no particular reason why you should have a seven-day break. As long as you don't stop for more than seven days, you can decide this for yourself. Remember, though, you don't have this option with progestin-only products.

If you use contraception that only contains progestin, for example an implant, hormonal IUD, or estrogen-free contraceptive pills, you won't get the side effects from estrogen detailed earlier. Nor will you have any of the positive effects of estrogen, such as clearer skin and control over your period. Progestin can actually cause skin breakouts and, in some cases, increased hair growth.

Perhaps the most important side effect that all women experience when they use progestin-only methods of contraception is a change in bleeding. This is quite harmless, but some people find it a nuisance. The changes vary according to the person and the type of progestin contraception used. You can't know how you'll react until you've tried it. Some women stop having periods entirely, while others may have more frequent light bleeding or irregular bleeding. Most have lighter bleeding than before, but it may last either more or fewer days. Once you've been using the contraceptives for three to six months, things tend to stabilize and you're able to recognize your unique pattern.

Despite the changes in bleeding that often occur with the implant and the hormonal IUD, these are still the two contraceptive methods we most strongly recommend. They have the best Pearl Index scores and are therefore the most effective means of preventing pregnancy. The hormonal IUD also has incredibly low hormone doses compared with all the other forms of contraception. A common misconception is that the hormonal IUD supplies the body with more hormones because it works for several years, but that's not true. The hormone concentration in the blood from using the smallest hormonal IUD is actually so low that it's equivalent to taking one single mini pill *every other week*![38] Some people think the low hormonal concentration reduces the chance of side effects, but that has not been proven. Even so, it may be worth trying if you've had a lot of trouble with other forms of contraception.

THE RARE SIDE EFFECTS

At the bottom of the list of side effects on the patient information leaflet are the ones that cause a media frenzy a couple of times a year, because there's no better click bait than the fear of disease and death. Well, apart from sex perhaps. In case you're in any doubt about it, there is no conspiracy between doctors and pharmaceutical companies to threaten the lives of healthy young women with hormones. There's even been a study to test it! A bunch of researchers from Harvard followed 120,000 women for thirty-six years to research the long-term effects of taking the Pill. They concluded that Pill users die just as often (or just as rarely, if you like) and from the same causes as women who don't use hormonal contraception.[39] In any case, we can strike death off our list of concerns related to the Pill.

BLOOD CLOTS

Although extremely rare, the use of contraception containing estrogen does have the risk of serious side effects that we need to talk about. The one that generally attracts the most attention is blood clots.

Blood clots occur when our blood coagulates, creating one or several lumps in a blood vessel. The lumps stop the flow of blood in this vessel—most commonly in the large veins in the legs and the pelvis. Veins, as opposed to arteries, are the blood vessels that carry blood from your organs and extremities back to the heart. Doctors call this deep vein thrombosis.

The reason we can get blood clots in our legs is that it's hard work for the blood to beat gravity when it's being dispatched back to the heart. The blood relies on assistance from contractions in the muscles to get up speed, like a pump. When we sit still for long stretches, such as on a plane journey, the blood may flow too slowly. In rare cases it may begin to coagulate. If you get a blood clot in your leg, you'll notice it swelling up and becoming red and painful.

The main reason why people are afraid of blood clots in the leg is that parts of the clot may come loose. Then they'll be swept away with the bloodstream back to the heart and onward, out into the lungs. Since the blood vessels in the lungs have a smaller gauge, the clot can get stuck there, causing respiratory problems. This is known as a pulmonary embolism. Although it can be serious, it is rarely fatal. One sign of having a blood clot in your lungs is if you experience sudden stabbing pains in your chest, which worsen when you breathe in. We all get small pains in our chest now and again, usually owing to tenderness in the muscles between our ribs, but the pains caused by a pulmonary embolism don't go away. At the same time, you may get short of breath and develop a cough. If you suspect you have a blood clot, it's important to go to the ER or an urgent care center for treatment ASAP.

As you've already learned, different contraceptives contain different hormones. Only contraceptives that contain estrogen increase the risk of blood clots. This includes regular pills, the contraceptive patch, and the vaginal ring. As we mentioned in the section about risk, the risk of blood clots rises two to four times when you're using combined contraceptives. The reason why we say two to four is because it depends on which type you're using. Of the estrogen-based contraceptives available today, the ones containing the levonorgestrel type of progestin involve the lowest chance of blood clots. There are several different types of pills containing levonorgestrel on the market in the United States: Alesse, Levlen, Levora, Nordette, and Ovranette. If you're going to use contraceptive pills for the first time, we recommend one of these.

Some women shouldn't use estrogen-based contraceptives at all, because they have a significantly increased risk of blood clots. The most important group are women with genetic disorders that affect the blood's ability to coagulate, for example a condition known as the Leiden mutation. This is why the doctor asks you whether your parents or siblings have had a blood clot when you're going to start using combined contraception.

As we mentioned earlier, the risk of healthy young women getting blood clots is incredibly small, regardless of whether they use estrogen-based contraception or not. If 100,000 women take the Pill, somewhere between forty and one hundred will suffer blood clots over the course of a year's use. If they hadn't been using the Pill, between twenty and fifty would still have gotten blood clots.[40*] It isn't true that the estrogen in contraceptive pills is more dangerous than the "natural" estrogen in the body. Pregnant women who

---

*   The numbers vary from study to study and depending on which age group and population type are being studied. The underlying risk of blood clots rises significantly with an increase in age and weight, and among smokers.

produce lots of estrogen are at greater risk of blood clots than users of contraceptive pills. For comparison, up to two hundred out of 100,000 women have blood clots while they are pregnant or in the period after giving birth.[41]

In other words, the likelihood of having a blood clot is greater if you have an unplanned pregnancy than if you are using contraceptive pills. The natural increase in hormones your body undergoes as a result of pregnancy is much more substantial than the increase we cause in order to prevent a pregnancy. This is one of the most important reasons why we should accept a slightly increased risk of blood clots when using contraceptive pills. It is, to put it simply, much more dangerous to become pregnant.

STROKE AND HEART ATTACK

Other serious side effects of estrogen-based contraceptives are stroke and heart attack. These are diseases that affect the arteries, i.e., the blood vessels that carry oxygen-rich blood from the heart to our organs. When this blood stream stops, whether because of a blood clot or a burst blood vessel, the tissue connected to the blood vessel can die due to lack of oxygen. This means that a part of the heart dies. Obviously, the consequences of such damage can be considerable.

A study in which all Danish women were examined between 1995 and 2009 found that the risk of stroke and heart attack was around twice as high among users of estrogen-based contraceptive pills.[42] However, remember the difference between relative and absolute risk: Although doubling the risk sounds dramatic, these are diseases that rarely affect young women. Even with twice the risk, the likelihood that you'll have a stroke is minimal.

To illustrate this we'll go back to the same study. Of the 100,000 women who used contraceptive pills for a year, around twenty had a stroke and ten had a heart attack. This included all types of Danish women who used contraceptive pills: obese and thin, smokers and nonsmokers, old and young. If it had only examined healthy young women, the risk would have been even lower.

Some women shouldn't use estrogen-based contraceptives in order to minimize the risk of stroke and heart attack. This applies to smokers over thirty-five, women with high blood pressure or heart disease, and those who have had diabetes for more than twenty years. Another group that should not use estrogen-based contraceptives is women who suffer migraines with aura. If, however, you have migraines *without* an aura, it's fine for you to use estrogen-based contraception as long as you're under thirty-five.

If you're exposed to too many risk factors that can lead to a stroke and heart attack—for example obesity, high cholesterol, and smoking—your doctor may advise you to choose another form of contraception to be on the safe side. Long story short, if you're young and healthy, there's no need to worry about stroke and heart attack even if you use estrogen-based contraception.

CANCER

In some circles there are still people who believe that contraceptive pills are carcinogenic. Let's start off by stressing the fact that using contraceptive pills and other hormonal contraception does not increase the likelihood that you will suffer from cancer over the course of your life.[43] In fact, several things indicate that, on the whole, contraceptive pills reduce the risk of cancer.[44] They seem to *protect* against cancer in the bowel, bladder, endometrium, and ovaries. Many of these types of cancer are common among women.

The use of contraceptive pills may protect against ovarian cancer for thirty years after you've stopped taking the pills.[45] If this figure is correct, researchers think that contraceptive pills will prevent 30,000 cases of ovarian cancer worldwide every year in the coming decades. Population-based studies indicate that contraceptive pills prevent cancer of the endometrium in the uterus for at least fifteen years and that the risk of acquiring this form of cancer is almost halved in comparison with women who have not used hormonal contraception.[46] Some researchers have delivered the message clearly: Contraceptive pills prevent gynecological cancer, and this positive side effect outweighs all the negative effects.[47]

However, it seems that contraceptive pills may somewhat increase the risk of cervical cancer. The best study that has been done in this area showed that ten years' use of contraceptive pills would increase the incidence of cervical cancer from 3.8 to 4.5 per 1,000 women.[48] The risk increased the longer you used contraceptive pills, but fell again once you stopped. Ten years after you stopped taking the pill, the risk was at the same level as before you began.

The problem is that it isn't possible to say for certain that the contraceptive pill itself increases the risk of cancer, because women who use it are also more prone to infection by HPV—that is, the virus that causes cervical cancer. It is easier to become infected with the virus because many women become more relaxed about using condoms with new partners when they're taking hormonal contraception. It has also been found that women using this kind of contraception have more sex than women who don't—after all, that's why they're using contraceptives in the first place.

Breast cancer is the last form of cancer that people wonder about when it comes to links with the contraceptive pill. We know that some types of breast cancer are "hormone sensitive"—meaning that they like estrogen, which they need in order to grow. Combined contraceptive pills contain estrogen, of course, and that might lead you to think that estrogen-based hormonal contraceptives help "feed" this type of cancer.

Luckily, that's not really how it works. Most major studies that have looked at breast cancer and the use of contraceptive pills haven't found any link, with a few exceptions. Individual studies have found a slightly increased risk between women who used the first high-dosage contraceptive pills in the 1960s and 1970s. However, experts think today's contraceptive pills and other combined products contain such low hormone doses that there's little likelihood they affect the risk of breast cancer.[49]

To sum up: Contraceptive pills and other combined products appear to protect women against a number of both common and serious types of cancer. This is something to take into account when you're looking at the overall picture for hormonal contraception. Unfortunately, these kinds of important, positive side effects get too little attention in the media compared to the rare, dangerous side effects.

WHAT WE'RE NOT SURE ABOUT

If you've read the patient information leaflet that comes with your contraception, perhaps you're surprised that we haven't mentioned two important side effects: mood swings and reduced sexual desire. It's not because we think they're unimportant—quite the opposite. The thing is that these are the side effects researchers are most uncertain about. And yet these two possible side effects are the ones that have been gaining increasing attention among women in recent years, so we think they deserve thorough consideration.

Natural sex hormones influence areas in the brain that are involved in regulating both mood levels and sexual desire. It's a well-known fact that women's moods can change according to the hormonal swings of the menstrual cycle. Some women find they're especially turned on around ovulation.[50, 51] It has even been observed that women are more unfaithful around ovulation![52]

With this in mind, it isn't so odd to think that contraceptives, which alter the sex hormone balance, might also have an effect on the psyche and sexual desire. Broad agreement has gradually emerged among women and many doctors that hormonal contraception can cause mood swings, irritability, and, in the worst case, depression. Mental and other nonspecific side effects are among the reasons women most commonly cite for giving up on contraceptive pills.[53, 54, 55]

Despite this agreement among women, researchers are struggling. Several studies have tried to prove that hormonal contraception has a negative effect on a woman's moods, without success. There may be several possible explanations for this.

FIRST POSSIBLE EXPLANATION: THE RESEARCH ISN'T GOOD ENOUGH

An incredible amount of research has been done into contraceptive pills. Over 40,000 articles have been written in the last few decades. The problem is that many of the studies are of poor quality, especially those dealing with side effects. Despite this, it's unlikely that side effects of hormonal contraception have been overlooked or understated. This might seem odd, but the "bad" studies are precisely the ones in which you find the most side effects. Most of the few good studies that have been undertaken tend instead to show few or no side effects. As a result, the many bad studies we have of the side effects of contraceptive pills contribute to an exaggerated idea of the scale and seriousness of these side effects.[56]

The thing that makes these studies faulty is that they've often taken women using hormonal contraception and asked them about side effects without controlling the findings against women who aren't using hormonal contraception. When researchers do that they can't actually draw any conclusions, because it's highly possible that all they've done is measure how common these symptoms are in the general population.

Imagine, for example, that 10 percent of all women have a headache once a month but aren't particularly concerned about it. If somebody were to ask them how often they had a headache, they'd have to guess. Then they take part in a study in which they will take contraceptive pills every day and keep a journal of all possible side effects. So in this study, one in ten will automatically report a headache, even though it has nothing to do with the contraceptive pills. This will not be discovered because there's no comparison with women who don't use contraceptive pills. Instead, it will seem as if the contraceptive pills cause the headache. These kinds of studies are common, and this is where hormonal contraception has most often been found to have effects on the psyche and sexual desire.

In medicine there's one kind of study that is considered to be the best, i.e., the absolute gold standard. Naturally, it has a fancy name: a randomized controlled study. This involves a group of people randomly divided into groups of those who do and those who do not receive a treatment. Those who do not receive treatment are the control group. Ideally, the study should also be blind, i.e., the patients (and preferably the doctor and researcher, too) don't know which treatment they're receiving. Only in studies like this is it possible to say anything about causal links, i.e., prove whether or not a medication is the cause of a given symptom.

As far as we know only four such randomized controlled studies have so far been carried out exploring contraceptive pills and nonspecific side effects such as mood changes.* Two of them found no significant difference in mood changes between those who did and didn't receive the pills.[57, 58] One study found that contraceptive pill use led to an improvement in symptoms of depression.[59]

In the last study, which looked at women from Edinburgh and Manila, a reduction in depressive symptoms was found among the women who received mini pills, while those who were given both placebo and contraceptive pills had a minimal increase in depressive symptoms.[60]

The exception is a small Swedish study. A group of researchers in Uppsala invited a group of women who had previously experienced psychological side effects from contraceptive pills to take part in a placebo-controlled study.[61] One half of the patients were given contraceptive pills and the other half were given sugar pills, without knowing which group they were in. The study found that, on average, those who received contraceptive pills experienced greater mental deterioration than those who did not. In addition, images were taken of the women's brains as they looked at photographs intended to evoke feelings. Changes in activity in parts of the brain

---

* One weakness of these studies is that they were carried out on groups who were using hormonal contraception for reasons other than to avoid getting pregnant, for example, because they had problems with acne or severe menstrual pains. Consequently, it's conceivable that these women are different from other women who use hormonal contraception and that this affects the results. For example, might women who have more problems with acne be more depressed?

that we know work with our feelings were observed among some of the women on contraceptive pills.

However, there is one big BUT here: This result applied to only one third of the pill users. Two out of three of the women taking contraceptive pills experienced *no* mental deterioration or changes in brain activity while taking the contraceptive pills, even though, by their own account, they tended to react adversely to hormonal contraception. These findings may indicate that contraceptive pills have a genuine negative effect on the psyche of a small group of women. But this applies to many fewer women than the number who *feel* this to be the case. That brings us to the next possible explanation: the power of chance.

SECOND POSSIBLE EXPLANATION: THE POWER OF CHANCE

We humans come equipped with a brain that likes to impose order and systems on the world around us. We try to sort our sometimes-chaotic environment by drawing connections between events even when connections don't exist. If two events are linked in time, we draw the conclusion that one caused the other. For example, you start taking contraceptive pills and three months later you suddenly notice you're a bit down. It must be because of the contraceptive pills, right? After all, you've never experienced a rough patch before as far as you recall.

But the Pill need not be the reason at all. Depression is a surprisingly common complaint in the population. Roughly one in five women experience clinical depression over the course of their lives,[62] and many more experience depressive feelings and thoughts. Depression is an illness with many complex causes. Personality type, biological changes in the brain, heredity, and life problems can all play a role. Because so many elements are involved it's rarely possible to point to a single concrete cause.

Depression, mood changes, and irritability are such common phenomena in the population that this is likely to be a trick of chance. If, in addition, you've heard that contraceptive pills can cause mood changes and depression, it's even more likely you'll draw this conclusion, given the nocebo effect we spoke about earlier (pages 158–9). Rumors of mood changes spread like wildfire among female friends on Internet forums, and suddenly you start to see your own experiences in a new light.

This theory is supported by many large population-based studies.[63] In Finland, Australia, and the United States, studies of this kind have resulted in negative findings. The Australian study followed 10,000 women for three years. There was no difference in the frequency of depressive symptoms between those who did and didn't use contraceptive pills. In addition, the study found that the longer women had used contraceptive pills, the less likely they were to have depressive thoughts.[64] The American study followed 7,000 women from 1994 to 2008. Here, in fact, the study found that women who used contraceptive pills had fewer depressive symptoms and were less likely to have attempted suicide in the last year than women who did not use hormonal contraception.[65] The Finnish study revealed similar results: Women who used hormonal contraception were simply *less* depressed than other women.[66]

The problem with these studies is, of course, that there may be underlying differences between women who use contraceptive pills and those who don't. It may be the case that all women who experience a deterioration in their moods stop taking contraceptive pills, while the ones who continue to take them are the ones who don't have negative reactions. In this way a negative effect may potentially be masked.

Given this criticism, researchers in Copenhagen carried out a gigantic population-based study of one million Danish women aged between fifteen and thirty-four, whom they followed from 2000 to 2013.[67] This study found that the use of contraceptive pills and other hormonal contraception was linked to an increased risk of needing antidepressants or receiving a diagnosis of depression compared with those who did not use hormonal contraception.

The effect appeared to be greatest among the youngest girls, aged between fifteen and nineteen, while the risk fell markedly once they hit twenty and continued to decrease as they grew older. Women over thirty experienced almost no increase in the use of antidepressants or the incidence of depression while using hormonal contraception. The researchers think the brain becomes less sensitive to hormone fluctuations as people age.

This study also observed that the risk of depression and the use of antidepressants became steadily lower the longer women spent on hormonal contraception. The risk was seen to be greatest after six months' use, after which it began to fall again. After four years on hormonal contraception there was no difference between users and non-users when it came to the risk of depression.

The researchers also found differences between different forms of contraception. Contraceptive pills appeared to give the lowest risk of use of antidepressants, whereas, for example, mini pills, the vaginal ring, and long-acting methods of contraception were linked to a greater risk. Although it's impossible to say anything for certain based on just one study, this underscores why women should have a low threshold for switching their method of contraception if they experience adverse side effects. There's variation among the side effects that different methods of contraception give women, so it's important to try multiple options if one isn't working.

Having said that, we advise some caution when interpreting this study. There has already been a lot of fear-mongering in Denmark warning women against hormonal contraception with a claim that taking it leads to depression. Believe it or not, you can't actually claim that on the basis of this study. What the study shows is that more girls who use hormonal contraception start taking antidepressants than those who don't use hormonal contraception. Nobody has proved that the hormonal contraception is the *cause* of the depression. This is an important distinction. In order to be able to say anything about causal links you have to use totally different research methods: randomized controlled studies. As we've already discussed, the few such studies that do exist have not shown anything approaching the same results. The Danish study is a solid piece of research that will probably lead to further serious investigation in the field, but until we have more studies showing the same results, we cannot conclude that hormonal contraception causes depression in certain women.

There's no getting away from relative versus absolute risk, either. Some newspaper articles about the Danish study reported that teenage girls have an 80 percent higher risk of depression. This sounds incredibly frightening, almost as if you're guaranteed to become depressed if you start taking the pill in high school. The truth is quite different. Every year, one in one hundred teenage girls in Denmark who are *not* using hormonal contraception are prescribed antidepressants for the first time. For comparison, 1.8 in 100 of those who do use hormonal contraception are prescribed antidepressants. *So we're talking about an increase of less than one extra person.* Ninety-eight of the girls using hormonal contraception don't seek treatment for depression and one girl would have sought treatment no matter what. These are the figures you should keep in mind, not alarming headlines about 80 percent increases. Once there's a proper presentation of facts on the table, you can make an informed choice about whether you still think this is reason enough not to start using hormonal contraception. We won't argue with you then.

We've introduced a lot of studies and presented contradictory results. We're aware that it may be difficult to digest all of this. Even so, we think it's possible to draw one important conclusion from these studies: Hormonal contraception can't possibly have a major negative effect on the psyche of most women. If such a side effect does exist, it applies to a minority of women who are, for one reason or another, prone to react adversely to the hormones. We hope to become better informed about who these women are in the future. Perhaps it's worth exercising caution if a lot of people in your family have been struggling with depression or if you have had depressive tendencies yourself in the past.

For the rest of us, it's time to stop worrying—and perhaps to take it with a grain of salt when we hear stories about awful psychological side effects from hormonal contraception.

* * *

We use hormonal contraception to be able to have as much care-free sex as we want, but what if hormonal contraception makes sex uninteresting? Is it true that contraceptive pills kill sexual desire? Many women seem to think so. In a Swedish survey almost 30 per-cent of women using hormonal contraception thought that one of its side effects was reduced sexual desire.[68]

The largest systematic review of hormonal contraception and sexual desire was carried out in 2013.[69] It combined the findings of thirty-six studies involving a total of 13,000 women, 8,000 of whom used contraceptive pills. Most of the women found that their sexual desire was unchanged (64 percent) or even increased (22 percent) after they started using contraceptive pills. Several studies observed an increase in sexual desire while taking contraceptive pills; this is believed to be because contraception eliminates anxieties about pregnancy—a passion killer for women the world over. As we dis-cussed earlier, sexual desire is simply a function of the balance between brake and accelerator. As such, researchers don't think that the hormones *directly* increase sexual desire. On the other hand, 15 percent of women experienced reduced sexual desire while using hormonal contraception. We can't say for certain whether the hor-mones are to blame.

What is known, however, is that the levels of active testoster-one in the body are reduced when using hormonal contraception. As we know, testosterone is the male hormone par excellence, but we women also produce a small dose of it. Bodybuilders who take testosterone to increase the size of their muscles often experience increased interest in sex (often with the tedious combination of micro-penis and poor-quality sperm). Could it be that women on hormonal contraception experience the flip side of this: that we lose our desire because of having too *little* testosterone?

Testosterone reduction occurs to varying degrees in different women and is also dependent on the type of contraception we use. Hormonal contraception contains different progestins, with dif-ferent effects on testosterone. Those containing drospirenone, like Yasmin, reduce testosterone levels. That may lead to less acne but also, perhaps, to reduced sexual desire. The levonorgestrel progestin contained in Loestrin, Ortho-Novum, and the hormonal IUD, however, has a more similar effect to testosterone and is therefore less likely to cause reduced sexual desire.

The problem with the testosterone theory is that no clear connection has been seen between the testosterone level in the blood and the degree of sexual desire experienced. Some women with relatively high testosterone levels struggle with low sexual desire, while other women with low testosterone don't have any issues. It's evidently not the case that sexual desire is proportional to testosterone levels. Even so, people have tried giving women testosterone to increase sexual desire—but without achieving any miraculous effects.* On average, they had one extra "satisfying sexual event" a month (they're great at talking dirty in the research world).[70]

Still, there's a lot we don't know about female sexuality. We may never find a good answer when it comes to the impact of hormonal contraception on sexual desire. It's a difficult topic to research because there's no good measure—or definition—for what desire actually is. And desire is influenced by so many factors in life that it's impossible to separate what is caused by contraceptive pills from the effects of a fading love affair.

As you've probably grasped already, the world of research is full of uncertainty. What we can say, however, is that there's little to suggest that hormonal contraception has a strongly negative effect on sexual desire in most women.[71]

It's possible your contraception may have reduced your libido, but it's not the most likely explanation. It's much more common for

---

*   The testosterone supplement was primarily tried out on postmenopausal women or women whose ovaries had been removed after cancer. Little is known about the long-term risk of testosterone use, and if a woman becomes pregnant while she's taking testosterone, the fetus may be damaged. In one of the few randomized studies on younger women (aged thirty-five to forty-six) the testosterone supplement was found to have little or no effect on sexual desire. However, the placebo effect was high.

sexual desire to ebb over the course of a relationship or for stress to rob us of the energy we need for sexual excitement.

Our advice, before you throw away your pills or make an appointment to have your contraceptive implant removed, is to assess whether there are other aspects of your life that may be contributing to your reduced sexual desire. You can also try to switch to a method of contraception containing a different progestin.

TIME FOR A HORMONE DETOX?

Sex is not a constant benefit for most of us. When you're in a steady relationship, perhaps you have sex several times a week; but then it ends and your single life is anything but an episode of *Sex and the City*. You begin to feel like an elephant on the savannah, searching for water at the height of the dry season. Your contraceptive pills become a bitter daily reminder of your involuntary celibacy and seem to taunt you from the bathroom cabinet: "Ha! You won't be getting any today either!"

At the same time, perhaps you've heard that hormones aren't good for you, that they're unnatural substances.[72] Why subject your body to sinister hormones when you're not even getting sex as compensation? You might think to yourself: *Let this period of being single be a time for detox, cleansing, and health! Time for a break from hormones!*

Stop right there. This isn't as smart as it sounds. If you've found a hormonal contraceptive that works for you, it's silly to stop just because you've become single. Most people who start taking hormonal contraception have certain side effects at the outset, but these usually pass or become milder after several months. The body adjusts to a new hormonal balance and settles down. When you stop, it'll take time for your body to return to a new balancing point, and you'll have exactly the same side effects again the next time you start.

Blood clots are, in fact, the main reason we don't recommend taking a break from hormonal contraception. Some studies indicate that the risk of blood clots is greatest in the first months after you start taking contraceptive pills, and decreases sharply over time.[73] If you use contraceptive pills on and off every time you meet a new partner, your body won't have time to return to balance. The result is that your dream guy won't just give you butterflies but also a higher risk of blood clots.

If blood clots are the dangerous but rare side effect of taking a hormone break, there's another one that's much more common. Lovers show up when you least expect them, and your doctor isn't available 24/7—so it's no surprise that taking a break from the pill often ends up giving you more of a detox than you'd bargained for. A nine-month detox, in fact. One in four women who take a six-month break from contraceptive pills end up having an unplanned pregnancy within half a year.[74] Quite naturally!

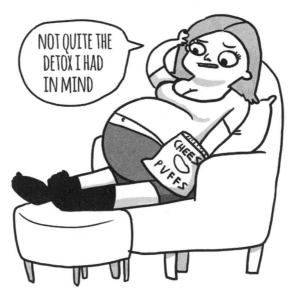

Some women are afraid that long-term use of hormonal contraception may make it difficult to get pregnant later in life. Luckily this is totally untrue, although it can take a few months for you to start ovulating again when you're on certain hormonal contraceptives. In fact, the likelihood of infertility is lower among women who've used hormonal contraception, because they appear to have a lower chance of suffering pelvic inflammations if they're infected with sexually transmitted diseases.[75] Unfortunately, there are women (and men) out there who can't have children for various reasons. The problem is that you won't know whether you're one of them until you stop using contraception and try to have a baby yourself. If you're thirty-five and fail to get pregnant, it's easy to blame the contraceptive pills you've been using since you were fifteen. Research shows, however, that contraceptive pills have no impact on women's fertility, whether they've been using them for one or ten years.[76] Age, however, does have a lot to do with it.

IN DEFENSE OF HORMONAL CONTRACEPTION

Recently, there's been a lot of public discussion about the troublesome aspects of hormonal contraception. We agree that it's a shame we don't have more contraceptive options to choose from and we'd very much like to see better contraception alternatives for men on the market. But the fact is that contraception is a necessary evil for women, because sex results in children. No matter how much we dislike it, this fact isn't going to go away—and of course we want to have sex.

Although the world of contraception is far from ideal, we believe that the many positive aspects of hormonal contraception are often overlooked. As such, we want to end this chapter by speaking up for hormonal contraception and offering a short speech in its defense.

Hormonal contraception is and will remain the most effective protection we have against pregnancy, alongside the copper IUD and sterilization. The harmless side effects that some women experience when using hormonal contraception are nothing compared to the problems most women experience during pregnancy: pregnancy-related pelvic girdle pain, massive amounts of discharge, swollen legs, hemorrhoids, and stretch marks—not to mention the dangerous, if rare, side effects. The danger of blood clots is much higher when you're pregnant than when you're using hormonal contraception.

Far too few people grasp the positive effects of hormonal contraception. We've already mentioned them, but there's no harm in summarizing them here:

- Hormonal contraception appears to offer protection against some of the most common forms of cancer in women: colorectal, ovarian, and endometrial cancer.
- Hormonal contraception reduces menstrual pain, leads to shorter and lighter bleeding, and decreases your chances of developing anemia, which is a major problem for many women.
- With combined contraception products, you can manage your bleeding so that it comes when you want it to.
- Hormonal contraception protects against pelvic infections—an important cause of infertility in women—by making the mucus plug in the cervix thicker and more impenetrable to bacteria.
- The chance of getting benign breast lumps—a cause of anxiety and surgical procedures for many young women—is reduced.
- Hormonal contraception is good at treating two common and troublesome female diseases: polycystic ovary syndrome and endometriosis.

It may be a good idea to remember this list when people portray hormonal contraception as women's mortal enemy. Because of the ways it has allowed women to control their fertility, their bodies, and their sexual choices, the contraceptive pill has been and continues to be one of the world's most vital discoveries when it comes to women's equality.

CONTRACEPTION GUIDE

Do you think it's difficult to choose contraception? With eleven types to choose from, it can feel overwhelming. But don't despair: We've prepared a contraception guide just for you. Since the most effective contraceptives are prescription-only, you'll have to make your choice in consultation with a doctor, midwife, or nurse, but it might be good to formulate some thoughts beforehand. Based on what's most important to you right now, you can choose the methods of contraception that suit you and find out which ones you'd be better off avoiding. You're probably concerned about a combination of the issues below, so it's a question of choosing the best alternative.

The Most Important Thing for Me Is to Avoid Pregnancy

If the most important thing for you is not to get pregnant, you should choose the most effective method of contraception there is—the so-called long-acting methods. At the top of the list you'll find the contraceptive implant and the hormonal IUD, closely followed by the copper IUD. Combined products, such as contraceptive pills, are also effective if you use them correctly.

Suitable: Long-acting contraception with a low Pearl Index: contraceptive implant, hormonal IUD, and copper IUD

Unsuitable: Methods with a high Pearl Index, especially those that are based on fertility awareness

I'm at High Risk for Blood Clots, Stroke, or Heart Attack

If you're at high risk for any of these diseases, you must avoid estrogen. You can still choose the methods of contraception that are best at preventing pregnancy—i.e., progestin-only products such as the contraceptive implant and the hormonal IUD. If you prefer taking contraceptive pills, there are also estrogen-free pills on the market in the United States, such as Microner, Camila, and Femulen.

Suitable: Estrogen-free methods: contraceptive implant, hormonal IUD, estrogen-free contraceptive pills, and copper IUD

Unsuitable: Combined products: combined pills, contraceptive patch, and vaginal ring

I Want Lighter Bleeding

Periods can be a pain, especially for women who have heavy, painful bleeding. Some women have it so bad that they develop anemia, or have to spend a week in bed each month because of the pain. If that sounds like you, it's handy to know that some methods of contraception can reduce bleeding. A general trait of all hormonal contraception is that the overall amount of blood is smaller. To find which one works best for you, you should experiment, by trial and error, in consultation with your doctor. The copper IUD often increases both bleeding and pain, so it isn't advisable for you.

Suitable: Hormonal contraception in general, particularly the hormonal IUD and combined products

Unsuitable: Copper IUD

I Want to Control When I Get My Period

As you may remember from the section called "Periods on Hormonal Contraception," contraception containing estrogen can be used to control your bleeding. Progestin-only products do not offer any menstrual control. If you're already using estrogen contraception without positive results, you can switch from a product with a low dose of estrogen to one with a slightly higher dose. You can, for example, switch from the Loestrin to the Ortho-Novum pill. This change doesn't increase your risk of blood clots.

Suitable: Combined products: combined pills, contraceptive patch, and vaginal ring

Unsuitable: Progestin products

I Have Trouble with Acne

If you struggle with acne, estrogen can help; in other words, you might consider combined products in consultation with your doctor. Progestin is often blamed for causing acne. If you're already using a combined product, you can try changing to another one containing a different progestin or a higher dose of estrogen. Remember that it can take up to three months for you to see any effect.

Suitable: Combined products: combined pills, contraceptive patch, and vaginal ring

Unsuitable: Products containing the same progestin you've already tried out

I Want to Hide My Method of Contraception from Other People

For some women it's important to hide the fact that they're using contraception from their partner or family. Some forms of contraception, such as the contraceptive implant, the copper IUD/hormonal IUD, or the contraceptive injection aren't visible, because they're inside your body. If you're concerned about hiding your contraceptive, you may wish to use a method that won't alter your pattern of bleeding, since changes in menstruation can affect your sex life or create noticeable changes in your routine. One alternative may be to use combined products or the copper IUD. These often give a regular cycle, although the total amount of blood may be altered. If it isn't a crisis for you to become pregnant, or if you live a very orderly life, you can also try the fertility awareness-based method to reduce the risk of pregnancy. But remember that one in four women who use such methods of contraception end up pregnant in the course of a year with typical use.

Suitable: Invisible contraception such as implant or hormonal IUD, or contraception that gives you a fixed cycle, such as combined products

Unsuitable: Depends on how you want to hide the method of contraception

I Want to Protect Myself Against Sexually Transmitted Infections

The condom is the only contraceptive method that protects you against STIs. We recommend that you use condoms in combination with another means of contraception until you and your partner have been tested for STIs.

Suitable: Condom and another contraceptive method combined

Unsuitable: Not using a condom

I'm Taking Other Medicines—So Can I Use Hormonal Contraception?

Medicines affect one another. If you're taking medicine for, say, epilepsy or mental illness, this can affect your contraception or vice versa. Your doctor will keep track of this. Perhaps she may give you a tailor-made solution.

Suitable: Your doctor will help you find the best solution if you're taking other medicines.

I Have Endometriosis

If you have endometriosis or suspect you might because of severe pains, hormonal contraception is the first step in your treatment. Since the aim is to stop having periods, you will not take breaks.

Suitable: Continuous use of combined products or insertion of a hormonal IUD

I Have Polycystic Ovary Syndrome or Extremely Irregular Periods

If you have fewer than four periods a year WITHOUT using hormonal contraception, you should start using hormonal contraception to expel the uterine lining at regular intervals—after discussing this with your doctor, of course. If menstruation is extremely rare, you can in fact experience excess growth of the uterine lining, which isn't good for you over the long term. Once you've had a couple of breakthrough bleedings on hormonal contraception, the problem is solved and you can start to skip bleeding as you wish.

Suitable: Combined products: combined pill, contraceptive patch, and vaginal ring

The Contraception I'm Using Reduces My Sexual Desire

It isn't certain whether hormonal contraception causes reduced sexual desire and, if so, which mechanisms are to blame. One theory is that this is caused by less active testosterone. Different types of progestin have different effects on testosterone. Those with drospirenone, such as Yasmin, reduce the testosterone level. That can reduce acne, and possibly also sexual desire. However, the levonorgestrel progestin found in Loestrin, Ortho-Novum, and the hormonal IUD has an effect that is more similar to testosterone and is therefore less likely to reduce your sexual desire.

Suitable: Products with the levonorgestrel progestin, such as Loestrin, Ortho-Novum, and the hormonal IUD, or hormone-free contraception such as the copper IUD

Less suitable: Products with the drospirenone progestin, such as Yasmin

PART 5: ABORTION

Abortion, the practice of intentionally terminating a pregnancy, provokes strong feelings. It's become a controversial issue worldwide in recent years, with many debating whose rights are primary: the pregnant woman's, or those of the unborn fetus.

For us, the woman's rights have the greatest weight—it's the woman who will undergo the physical and mental strain of pregnancy and birth. It is also often the woman who is left with the responsibility for care and provision of support. A child results in greater emotional, economic, and social upheaval for the woman, and the women who have the least to begin with are often the ones who are hit the hardest. It ought to be a woman's choice whether she wants to take on these burdens. There are no other areas of policy where it's acceptable to impose such considerable personal cost on a citizen to satisfy society's moral norms as when we oblige a woman to give birth to a child she doesn't want to have or is in no financial position to care for.

That said, it is reasonable to impose some limits on abortion. Most people agree that at some point in the pregnancy, the fetus is no longer a fetus but a child, with rights that outweigh the preferences and rights of the pregnant woman. Where that limit is set varies from country to country. In countries where abortion is legal and accessible, most abortions take place early in the pregnancy, while the rare late-term abortions that are carried out are often done so because of serious or life-threatening abnormalities in the fetus or to save the mother's life.

There are, for example, very different ways of regulating abortion—ranging from total prohibition in Chile and Malta, to

Norway, where women have a right to abortion on demand up to and including week twelve, to Canada, where there is no abortion law, but where abortion is considered to be a medical matter between a woman and her doctor. There are also major differences in the accessibility of abortion: It may be so expensive or offered in so few places that it is not a feasible option for many women, even though it isn't prohibited. For example, twenty-two states plus the District of Columbia in the United States have five or fewer abortion clinics.[1]

Regardless of your personal feelings about the question of abortion, it's indisputable that prohibiting or complicating access to abortion doesn't reduce the number of abortions. It's often the case that countries with the strictest legislation also have the highest incidence of abortions, while those with good access to legal abortion often have low abortion rates[2]—this is largely because countries with access to safe abortion also tend to provide better sex education and access to contraception. Throughout history and in every corner of the world women with unwanted pregnancies have taken matters into their own hands, despite threats of punishment and social ostracism—not to mention the risk of exposure to serious injury or death. The thought of giving birth to an unwanted child can be so unbearable that it outweighs the dangers and threats of legal prosecution.

Knitting needles, steep staircases, and poison are still last resorts for women in parts of the world where abortion is illegal or inaccessible. Every year, twenty million women feel obliged to undergo unsafe abortions—that's almost one in ten pregnancies worldwide. Of these women, 50,000 die unnecessary deaths.[3] Nearly seven million women require medical treatment for complications resulting from dangerous abortions.[4] Access to safe abortion would have spared them. Legal and safe abortion is, in other words, essential for safeguarding women's health. Prohibiting abortion doesn't save any potential children; it just harms desperate women.

That said, abortion is not an easy way out. Few women want to have an abortion or consciously use it as an alternative to contraception. It's often due to bad luck in the form of unprotected sex at the wrong time, contraceptive failure, poor access to modern contraception, or—in the worst case—assault and sexual violence. If the goal is to keep abortion figures low, the most effective measure is to ensure easily accessible, effective contraception, and to provide good sex education. Unfortunately, restrictive abortion laws often go hand in hand with poor access to precisely these aspects of health care. It's like an ostrich sticking its head in the sand and thinking the problem will go away just because it doesn't have to see it.

Regardless of whether you live in a country where abortion is easily accessible or not, it's good to know about how abortions are performed within the health system. Practices vary from country to country when it comes to how abortions are carried out—whether at a hospital or a specialized clinic, and what rules apply—but the methods are the same. If you find yourself in the position of having an unwanted pregnancy, it's good to be able to focus your thoughts on more important things than finding out practical details.

HOW FAR ALONG AM I?

A common source of confusion when it comes to abortion is how far along you are in the pregnancy. Many countries have abortion laws that involve time limits; for example, abortion on demand is allowed up to and including week twelve in many places. But when are you actually twelve weeks pregnant? You'd think it would be calculated from the date you had unprotected sex, but incredibly enough, that's not the case. Instead, it's calculated from the first day of your last period. This is because that's the last point in time you knew for sure that you weren't pregnant. Seen from this perspective, the law considers you to be "pregnant" for two weeks before you even had the intercourse that made you pregnant.

Before you have an abortion, most doctors will give you an ultrasound. A little probe, the thickness of two fingers, is inserted into your vagina to see how many weeks along you are. If the fetus in your uterus is longer than around 6.6 centimeters, for example, it is deemed to be more than twelve weeks old. The examination makes sense, because a lot of women have irregular periods or don't remember the date of their last period. The ultrasound examination is the legal answer to how far along you are, if there's any doubt about the matter.

TWO METHODS OF ABORTION

There are two ways of carrying out an abortion: with pills or with minor surgery. Abortion with pills is called a medical abortion, while the other method is called surgical abortion.

MEDICAL ABORTION

A medical abortion starts with you taking a pill, normally at a hospital or at a doctor's office. The pill contains a substance called mifepristone, which tricks the body into thinking you're no longer pregnant. All the complicated processes that make sure the fertilized egg grows into a fetus and then a baby come to a halt. The abortion has been set in motion, and although the process is not complete, you can't have second thoughts after taking the first pill—as a rule, the fetus will not develop any further in the normal way.

Once you've taken the pill, you have to wait one to two days before the abortion can be completed. It's perfectly normal to have mild nausea, light bleeding, and menstrual pains during this time, but otherwise, you can carry on with life as normal. Contact your doctor if you experience persistent fever, severe abdominal pain, fast heartbeat, prolonged heavy bleeding, or fainting. After roughly two days, the abortion must be completed. If you're a healthy woman who's been pregnant for less than nine to ten weeks, it's usually done at home. It's important, though, to have another adult with you, such as a friend or your partner, in case of complications—although complications are highly uncommon.

To complete the abortion, you insert four tablets of misoprostol in your vagina or place them under your tongue. In countries where abortion is illegal, it has gradually become more and more common for women to carry out abortions by obtaining misoprostol online or by other means. The pills cause the uterus to contract and squeeze out its contents—kind of like when you have your period, just that this time there's also a tiny fetus in your uterus that will come out along with the blood.

Once the abortion is underway, you'll have heavier bleeding than with a normal period. The blood that comes out will be clotted and red. If you're afraid of seeing the fetus, all we can say is that the earlier you have the abortion, the less of a chance there is that you'll see anything. Most abortions in Norway happen before the ninth week of pregnancy, when the fetus will be a 1.5-centimeter-long transparent tadpole surrounded by mucus and blood. Any pictures you've seen on the Internet of sweet little mini-babies are thoroughly misleading and designed to make women feel guilty about having an abortion.

For 95 to 98 percent of all women, the second part of a medical abortion is over in a few hours.[5] You should take painkillers, as ordered by your doctor, because it may hurt. If you still suffer severe pains, fever, or extremely heavy bleeding after an abortion, you should call your doctor or go to the ER. People often say that if you bleed through a heavy-duty nighttime pad in less than two hours, you should contact the doctor.

After the abortion, it is quite normal to experience light bleeding and feel some pain for two to three weeks. In that case, it's important to use pads and not tampons, in order to prevent infection. In addition, you should not have sex while you're bleeding. As long as you're bleeding, it means that the uterus is still getting rid of the remains of the pregnancy, and any bacteria that may find their way up the vagina can easily progress farther into your system. It isn't common to get infections after an abortion, but it's still important to take precautions.

Now and then you read horror stories in the media about women who had a medical abortion and discovered that they were still pregnant several months later. If you follow the instructions you get from your doctor, this is very unlikely. One in a hundred patients has been seen to remain pregnant after a medical abortion. You will be able to tell if this has happened because there will be no heavy bleeding after you've taken the misoprostol. In that case, you should contact your health care provider or clinic immediately. The pills you're taking terminate the pregnancy, and it isn't good to have the remains of it in your uterus. All women who have a medical abortion should take a pregnancy test a month later to ensure that the pregnancy is completely terminated. In addition, you should contact the clinic if your period has not returned four to six weeks after the bleeding stops.

SURGICAL ABORTION

A surgical abortion involves a slightly different process and must be carried out at a hospital or abortion clinic. In the United States, if you're going to be given anesthesia during the abortion, you'll be instructed not to have food or drink eight hours before the procedure. Many clinics do abortions using only local anesthesia. Outside of the United States, you'll usually be given pills in advance that cause the cervix to dilate, which can make the procedure less painful. Although this isn't common practice in the United States, you can request this medication from your doctor if you're worried about pain.

The operation itself lasts around ten minutes. After dilating the cervix, the doctor will access the uterus via the vagina and then the cervix. After that, she will suction out the fetus and the placenta using a small aspirator, and then she will gently scrape the uterine lining to ensure that everything has been removed. This procedure is often called D&C, or dilation and curettage. Following the abortion, you'll have to remain at the clinic for a few hours so that the doctor or nurse can check that everything's going well. After that, you can go home the same day.

As with a medical abortion, you may bleed and have pains for a while afterward. The same rules apply for sanitary pads and sex, and here, too, you should contact the clinic if you become unwell, bleed heavily, or don't start your period again within six weeks.

As with all surgery, there's a small risk of complications linked to anesthesia or the procedure itself. This includes damage to the uterus, bladder, or urinary tract. These very rare complications are the reason why medical abortion is recommended in many countries. It's always best to avoid an operation, but, all in all, surgical abortion carried out by health professionals is very safe. Many women prefer a surgical abortion to avoid the lengthier process involved in a medical abortion.

Some people may have heard that surgical abortion can make it more difficult to become pregnant later on. This impression stems from a rare condition called Asherman's syndrome, which can come about if the surgeon has to scrape out a great deal of tissue from the uterus and ends up damaging the deepest layer of the uterine lining. Then you may get uterine scarring and adhesions, which could make it difficult to get pregnant later. Abortion providers take care to avoid this. In other words, it's unlikely that an uncomplicated curettage will have any effect on your chances of becoming pregnant later. But the more times you have curettage, the greater the risk.[6] This is one of the reasons why abortion should never be used as a means of contraception.

Discovering that you have an unplanned pregnancy can be a shocking experience. Pregnancy can set in motion many emotional processes that you may not have been prepared for. If that happens, it's good to have somebody to talk to. All health care professionals have a duty of confidentiality and can offer you guidance through the process, whatever you might choose to do—whether you end up having an abortion, keeping the child, or choosing adoption. It's also sensible to talk to your partner, friends, and family to seek advice and care, whatever you choose to do.

PART 6: TROUBLE DOWN BELOW

Our genitals are just like the other parts of our body. As long as everything's working right, we don't give them much thought. As soon as something starts to go wrong, though, it can become an all-consuming business. Any woman who's had a severe yeast infection, for example, or who's struggled with menstrual pains knows all about this. On days like those, we may curse the day we were born women. What wouldn't we give to exchange our monthly cramps for the occasional kick in the balls?

We're absolutely certain that most women will experience some kind of trouble down below over the course of their lives. Fortunately, most gynecological ailments are not life threatening, but we can't deny that some of them may cause serious reductions in quality of life. The world of medicine has fallen short in many aspects of female health and we can only hope that sometime soon this will change, that women's disease will be a prioritized field.

While writing this chapter, we found ourselves feeling uncertain about whether we might not end up creating more anxiety than necessary. By talking about rare and dangerous diseases whose symptoms are often vague, might we be exposing women to new and unnecessary concerns?

We hope and believe that's not the case. Remember that your body is always giving off small signals indicating well-being or ailments. We're supposed to notice the fact that we are alive—we're not machines, after all. But some of us are more alert to these signals than others, and that can lead to health-related anxiety. We think the best medicine for this kind of anxiety is more knowledge. More knowledge can give you security, but scaring yourself silly by Googling vague, common symptoms can only make the terror worse. The trick is to distinguish between normal phenomena that we all experience now and then, and those that may be signs of something more serious.

In our work as sexual health writers, we've discovered that there's a remarkable lack of knowledge in the general public regarding common gynecological illnesses. A lot of women are struggling with diseases that those around them have never heard of, and they often feel lonely and mistrusted, as if they're making the whole thing up. Many don't know where to find help. For example, we'd never heard of endometriosis before we started studying medicine. But even so, one in ten women are walking around with this disease, and many are struggling to adapt their everyday life to the pain. That's not the way it should be. Imagine if one in ten men had to take a week off work each month because of excruciating pain in their balls. It would be a worldwide issue, covered in the curriculum at every school and debated in the upper tiers of government.

In other words, it's about time we spoke up about *our* problems. That's the only way we can ensure that people get the help they need. More resources should also be assigned to research into female diseases so that we can find effective treatments.

We'll start with the most common problems of all: bleeding disorders.

BLEEDING ABNORMALITIES—HIGH CRIMSON TIDE

Periods are a significant part of life for most women. From puberty until we are somewhere between the age of forty-five and fifty-five (more or less) our menstrual cycle follows an eternal circle, month after month. We are used to it being one of the reliably stable elements in our lives.

With that in mind, it's no wonder you get worried and confused when something happens to your period and the cycle is different from what you hear it *ought* to be. *Crisis*, you think—and you're not the only one. It's odd that changes in blood and mucus from your uterus should feel so alarming, but it's easy to believe something's wrong with the very core of your womanhood. Your thoughts get all tangled up in your head. *Is there something wrong with me? Will I be able to have kids ten years from now, as planned? Is it cancer? Is it a disease? Seriously—help!*

There are a lot of different types of bleeding abnormalities. They may involve pain, irregularity, problems with the amount of flow, or your period might simply stop. Let's discuss the most common ones.

WHEN YOUR PERIOD STOPS

One of the most common, and perhaps most frightening, things is when your period vanishes without a trace. Or *with* a trace. Sometimes you're left with trace bleeding, or "spotting," even though your usual menstrual bleeding has disappeared into thin air.

When your period stops for more than three months in the case of women who previously had regular periods, or nine months for those who were irregular, we call it *amenorrhea*.[1] All we mean by regular periods is that your menstrual cycle is equally long every time and that your period arrives on or about the same time every month, so that you can predict when it will come by using a menstrual calendar. *Amenorrhea*, from the Greek, means "without the monthly flow." And that's exactly what it is.

It's common for a woman's period to stop. As many as 8 percent of all women between sixteen and twenty-four experience this every year, and there can be different causes.[2] The first thing you need to think about is that your period stops when you're pregnant. *But I used a condom, didn't I*, you think, when you're three days late. You're not ready for kids right now, and the panic is close to the surface.

A pregnancy test at the right time can rule out pregnancy. Get tested if you're in any doubt. It's incredibly important to check whether you're pregnant if there's any possibility of it. Was there a contraceptive failure? A missed pill? Did you rely on withdrawal or a calendar method? Buy a pregnancy test—it's reliable three weeks after unprotected sex or contraceptive failure. If you haven't had sex or if you use safe contraception that can't be used incorrectly—e.g., the contraceptive implant or the hormonal IUD—there's another issue. There are most likely other reasons why your monthly bleeding has vanished.

One rare but funny cause of amenorrhea is travel. We don't know why it happens, but long plane journeys, especially if you cross several time zones, can mess with your menstrual cycle, causing the bleeding to come at the wrong time, as if it had jet lag.

Two much more common reasons for skipped periods are weight changes and excessive exercising. It's difficult to define just how large the weight change must be or how much you need to exercise for this to happen. Professional athletes often have amenorrhea, but you don't have to be a professional to exercise your period away. An anorexia diagnosis based on the strictest criteria requires your periods to have stopped, although that doesn't mean you have to have anorexia if your period stops due to weight changes.

Mental stress may also alter your period, although women differ widely in how susceptible their cycle is to these changes. One way of thinking about it is that your period is a sign that you have energy to spare. For you to become pregnant, your body should be strong enough to bear it. Pregnancy is a strain and if, for one reason or another, you lose the energy reserves you need to give birth to a child, your period might stop to protect you from a pregnancy for which you're not ready. Everything's connected. Body, mind, and period are no exception. So if your period is unexpectedly late, it might be because you've got too much to do at school this semester, or because you've been exposed to major psychological traumas such as an accident or a death in your family. Also, during the first couple of years after you start having periods, it's absolutely normal to have irregular menstruation. That includes your period stopping for a while. It takes time for your hormones to settle into balance and for ovulation to happen on a monthly basis. It'll sort itself out.

It may also be good to remember how contraception affects periods. Progestin products such as the hormonal IUD, the contraceptive injection, the estrogen-free pill, and the implant often cause periods to stop over time. This is completely normal and doesn't mean there's anything wrong. The bleeding that comes when you use contraception is not a normal period but what we call "withdrawal bleeding." Unlike a regular period, it's not a sign of having energy reserves. If you stop bleeding as a result of hormonal contraception, you don't have amenorrhea.

That being said, if your period disappears for a long time and you don't know why, a trip to the doctor is always a reasonable response. There are a number of illnesses that can lead to loss of menstruation. These include, among others, polycystic ovary syndrome, metabolic diseases, and pituitary adenomas.

IT HURTS!

More than half of us suffer from severe menstrual pains: unpleasant, cramp-like aches in our lower abdomen. As long as you've ruled out the possibility that the cramps have any special cause—e.g., an illness that causes more severe menstrual pains—this is known as primary dysmenorrhea. If the cramps have an underlying cause, they are called secondary dysmenorrhea. Dysmenorrhea means "painful menstruation." Some women also have pains in the small of their backs, their thighs, or their vaginas. The pain is worst in the first few days of menstruation and is often accompanied by other ailments, such as nausea, vomiting, and diarrhea. Up to one in six women suffer such severe pain that they have to take a couple days off work or school every month.[3]

Menstrual cramps are caused by contractions of the uterus. That little hollow bundle of muscles clenches itself tight toward the end of each cycle to push out the endometrium, the inner uterine lining that emerges as menstruation.

The uterus is strong—maybe too strong for its own good. It squeezes so tight that it can't catch its breath, and that hurts! Of course your uterus doesn't actually breathe—only your lungs do that—but all the cells in your body need a continuous supply of oxygen. Without that, they'd suffocate. The oxygen is carried in the bloodstream and what happens during menstrual cramps is that the uterus clenches its muscles so tightly that it shuts off its own blood supply in the process. It's that eager to get rid of the old endometrium! The pain you feel is caused by lack of oxygen in the tissue.

But hold on a minute—haven't you heard about something like this before? If you work in health care or if, for example, you have a grandparent with a condition called angina pectoris, this might sound unmistakably familiar. Indeed, pain caused by lack of oxygen is exactly what people get when the blood vessels in their heart are blocked. They might experience chest pains during physical activity. If Granddad goes up the stairs, his heart needs more oxygen, but his narrow vessels can't manage to transport the blood quickly enough. Then the heart suffers "hypoxic pain." Exactly the same thing happens in your uterus when it's grinding away to shed the endometrium.

You can also get chest pains from a heart attack. In that case, there's so little oxygen that part of your heart suffocates and dies. If you're starting to feel worried now, let us reassure you: menstrual pains aren't the same as a heart attack—they're not dangerous! You won't lose parts of your uterus as a result of the cramps, although it's interesting to realize that lack of oxygen is the cause of the pain in both cases. It isn't the same, but it's similar.

So why is it so painful for some people, while others think periods are a breeze?

The answer is thought to lie in how active your enzymes are. Enzymes are small proteins that ensure all the chemical processes in your body follow their proper course. One group, called COX enzymes, is involved in producing substances called prostaglandins. Among others, prostaglandins are the substances sometimes given to pregnant women to induce childbirth. They cause the uterus to contract, in turn causing the lack of oxygen we've just described.

Some experts think that women who have particularly painful periods have especially active COX enzymes.[4] As a result, they produce more prostaglandins than other women. This, in turn, results in stronger contractions of the uterus just when it's struggling to relax. The prostaglandins also make the nerves in the genital area hypersensitive to pain.

In case you've been wondering whether you have a low pain threshold or find people don't believe you when you describe your pain, here's a little comparison with childbirth that should shut most people up. It has been observed that the uterine contractions of women with dysmenorrhea can reach a pressure equivalent to 150 to 180 mmHg.[5] Perhaps that doesn't mean anything to you, but for comparison, the pressure during the pushing stage of childbirth is around 120 mmHg. During childbirth, women have three to four rounds of uterine contractions every ten minutes. During her period, a woman with dysmenorrhea may have between four and five such rounds. In other words, the pressure during awful cramps is at least as high as during birth and the pains come at slightly shorter intervals. Mercifully, for most women these horrible pains ease off over the years.

You can use painkillers for menstrual cramps, but it is important to use them correctly. Ibuprofen directly inhibits the COX enzymes, ensuring that fewer prostaglandins are produced. This is why ibuprofen and similar meds, known as NSAIDs ("nonsteroidal anti-inflammatory drugs"), are the most effective medication for menstrual pains. If you tend to have severe period pains, you should start taking ibuprofen a day before your period, or at least immediately when you notice the slightest sign of pain. After that you should take painkillers every six to eight hours in the first few days of your period without a break. Far too many people wait until it's really hurting before they take painkillers and unfortunately they are then much less effective because the prostaglandins have already been produced.[6]

Other than that, most forms of hormonal contraception have a positive effect on menstrual cramps. Contraceptives are also a more long-term solution, since you use them continuously.

Finally, it's important to point out that some people may have underlying causes for the pain. This is particularly true for women who find that the pain changes or increases suddenly or sneaks up on them over time. *It wasn't like this before.* This may indicate that you have knots of muscle in the uterus, known as fibroids, or endometriosis, in which extra uterine lining is produced outside the uterus. It's also possible to have worse cramps as a result of a copper IUD. If this applies to you, it's time to switch to another method of contraception.

If you experience sudden, severe pain, you might consider more serious, acute conditions. For example, it's possible for a pregnancy to develop outside the uterus. This can happen if the fertilized egg doesn't make its way down to the uterus as it should. Then the fetus begins to develop, say, in the fallopian tubes, where there isn't room for it. Pregnancy outside the uterus can manifest itself as severe menstrual pains, sometimes concentrated on one side. In that case, a trip to your urgent care clinic or ER is in order.

IRREGULAR PERIODS

In your first years of having periods, your last years of having periods, and when you're using hormonal contraception, it's normal for your periods to be somewhat irregular. It takes time for your cycle to stabilize after you start menstruating, and when you're on hormonal contraception you no longer have a normal period, because your cycle isn't the way it was before. With the exception of these situations, your cycle should stabilize, settling into a regular length of between twenty-one and thirty-five days. More or less. But if you've been having periods for several years and the bleeding is still (or suddenly becomes) as unpredictable as the plot of *Gone Girl*, you should pay attention.

Irregular bleeding can mean a variety of things. It may be spotting (small drops between each period), bleeding at unexpected times, or bleeding that happens after or in connection with sex. As well as stopping, your period may also be delayed or arrive unexpectedly as a result of stress, weight changes, or excessive exercise. Things like that influence our hormones. Other causes may be underlying illnesses, such as polycystic ovary syndrome or metabolic diseases.

Cervical cancer or STIs may cause the cervix to become tender and bleed slightly. If that happens, intercourse can trigger light bleeding during or after sex. Because of this, you should get bleeding associated with intercourse checked out by a doctor.

If you're using combined contraceptives (pills, contraceptive patch, or vaginal ring) and suffer from irregular bleeding, it may be a good idea to talk to your doctor or nurse. Many women find irregular bleeding stops when they switch to a product that contains more estrogen. There are two different doses of estrogen in contraceptive pills. For example, Loestrin is a low-dose pill, whereas Ortho Tri-Cyclen and Yaz contain higher doses. Otherwise, the pills are the same.

TOO MUCH BLOOD!

As you can see from the wide range of sizes and absorbencies available on the tampon shelf at the drugstore, your female friends won't necessarily bleed as much or as little as you. Women who bleed the least might only need to stick a tissue in their underwear to solve the problem. Others have to change their super-plus tampons every few hours and the fear of bleeding through makes them yearn for even higher absorbency levels—super-plus extreme.

Blood loss over the course of a cycle tends to vary a lot from one woman to the next, but the average is between 25 and 30 milliliters—-i.e., around the size of a single espresso at your local café. It's also within the norm to bleed a double espresso.[7]

Are you one of those women who's hooting with laughter now? *A single espresso? Over the course of the whole period? Ha ha—pathetic! A double a day at least!*

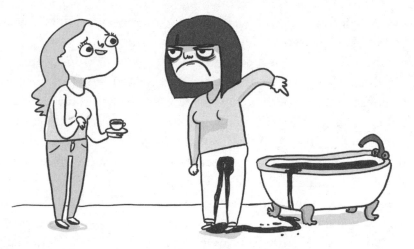

Some periods feel more like Lady Báthory's bathtub—the serial killer from Transylvania said to have bathed in the blood of virgins to stay young—than a chic shot at your local coffee shop. But no, nobody bleeds a whole bathtub's worth of blood over a single cycle, although it can seem that way when the blood charges through tampons, panties, and jeans and straight onto your best friend's white IKEA sofa. In fact, it would take approximately seven women's lifelong production of period blood to fill up a bathtub with a volume of around fifty gallons. Still, a lot of women have heavy enough periods that they end up becoming anemic and need to take iron supplements. Then they get sluggish and pale, often have headaches, and don't feel like doing any of the stuff they like. Periods can really make you lose your sparkle!

Menstrual bleeding is considered to be unusually heavy if either you bleed longer than eight days per cycle or the volume is over 80 milliliters[8]—so more than two and a half single espressos. Not exactly a bathtub, but a lot of blood all the same.

It's common for young girls to bleed more in the first few months or years after they start their periods. Things can improve over time and it's rarely a cause for concern. However, some girls have such heavy bleeding that it may be sensible to check that it isn't caused by an underlying disease. Certain blood disorders can in fact cause you to bleed more than other people—but this is rare.

The copper IUD is a common culprit when it comes to heavy bleeding. Many women find this contraceptive method works very well, but others experience an increase in menstrual bleeding and pain. This is particularly true for women who had heavy bleeding before getting the copper IUD. Combined contraceptives may be used to treat heavy bleeding, since they give you better control of it. Progestin products, like the hormonal IUD, which often eliminate your period entirely or substantially reduce the amount of blood, are also winners.

Women who've been having periods for a while and gradually start to have problems with heavy bleeding may have an underlying disease such as polycystic ovary syndrome (page 208), which messes with your hormones. The heavy bleeding can also be caused by fibroids, knots of muscle in the wall of your uterus (page 212).

ENDOMETRIOSIS—A UTERINE CARPETBAGGER

The pain of periods is something we women often take as a given, but some have such severe menstrual cramps that they have to put their whole life on hold. Several days a month they lie there, curled up on the sofa with heating pads, snacking on painkillers as if they were candy. If that's how it is for you, it's possible you may be suffering from something called endometriosis, a condition that affects around one in ten women. A third of those who struggle with this sort of pain in the lower abdomen and genitals have endometriosis.[9]* Of course, this does not apply to pain in the vulva itself, which we'll come back to later.

As you may have gathered from the name, endometriosis involves the endometrium, the mucous membrane that lines the inside

---

* It is difficult to know just how many people are affected, because many women don't have symptoms and the diagnosis can only be established through an operation.

of the uterus. This is the membrane that builds up every cycle as your uterus prepares to receive a fertilized egg, and is expelled from the uterus in the form of menstruation if you don't get pregnant. What's different when it comes to endometriosis is that those who suffer from it also have uterine lining *outside* their uterine cavity. In some cases, the uterine lining has gone astray in the muscle wall of the uterus, a condition known as adenomyosis.

It's not clear how this lining ends up outside the uterus. One leading theory is that the period has run the wrong way, i.e., it's gone up the fallopian tubes instead of out the cervix and ended up in the abdominal cavity. This happens to all women to a certain extent when they have their period, but it seems there are some susceptible women whose bodies can't manage to get it all cleaned up. When that happens, small groups of mucous membrane cells misunderstand where they belong, settling down in the pelvis, on the ovaries, in the gut, or other places in the abdomen.

Most often, these endometrial cells are found close to the internal sex organs, but in some very rare cases they can be found as far up as the sacs that surround the lungs. This has prompted some to wonder whether there may be other mechanisms causing endometriosis apart from periods gone astray. Perhaps there's a kind of stem cell—i.e., the cells that can become whatever cell they want to—that has developed in the wrong place? Or maybe cells from the uterine lining are transported in the bloodstream to other parts of the body? Hopefully we'll find a conclusive answer in the next few years.

The colonies of endometrium haven't forgotten where they come from, even though they've found a new home, carpetbaggers that they are. They behave as if they were living in the uterus—they react to the hormones in the menstrual cycle, just like ordinary endometrium do. Incredibly enough, this means that every month, you also have a mini-menstruation outside your uterus.

A misplaced period is not a popular event. The immune defenses put up a particularly stubborn fight when endometrium settles down in an otherwise quiet and orderly neighborhood, because the body has strict rules about what should happen where. When these endometrial colonies begin to bleed in a place where they don't belong, rebellion quickly follows. The new neighbors don't have a clue what's going on when they suddenly get hit by an unexpected shower of blood and, naturally enough, they call the police—our immune cells—which arrive at top speed to clean things up. The result is that you get an inflammation of the tissue surrounding the endometrial colony. And inflammation hurts.

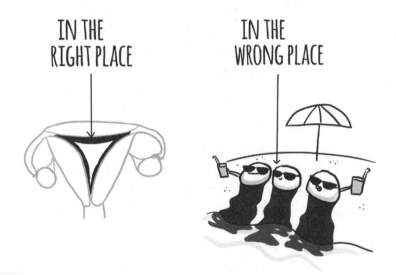

IN THE RIGHT PLACE

IN THE WRONG PLACE

Most people will find it difficult to distinguish these pains from severe but normal menstrual cramps, since the endometrial colonies are most often located close to the uterus, although some women will also find they have pain in odd places. For example, if the colonists have settled near the urinary tract, it may hurt to urinate, or if they're happiest in the rectum, defecating will be painful.

The one thing that all of these types of pain have in common is that they're cyclical—i.e., they follow a fixed pattern. They often come one or two days *before* menstruation and may continue for several days after it has ended. One way you can distinguish endometrial pain from ordinary menstrual cramps is that they usually develop gradually several years after you first start your periods, as if your menstrual cramps are steadily getting worse as you get older.

Some people do experience the pain from early in their teens, but this is less common. As a result, people don't tend to get diagnosed with endometriosis until they're over nineteen.

Over time, the monthly inflammations around the colony can cause scarring and adhesions inside the body. For example, the bladder may adhere to its neighbor, the uterus. These internal scars can cause chronic pain in the genital area. Many women with endometriosis also experience deep, stabbing pains during intercourse. The pain is in the lowest part of your abdomen, not in your vagina or vulva.

Another problem is that many women with endometriosis have difficulty conceiving. Endometriosis is responsible for around a quarter of all cases of involuntary childlessness.[10] We don't know exactly why people have problems with fertility. Scarring and adhesion can damage the fallopian tubes and the ovaries, but it looks as though other mechanisms are to blame, too, involving both the immune defenses and hormones. If you have endometriosis and you're struggling to get pregnant, artificial insemination may help.[11] Operations are available in addition to or instead of artificial insemination. Surgical removal of the colonies of endometrium outside the uterus has helped some women get pregnant, both naturally and through artificial insemination. The recommendation is that the operation should be carried out only once, and that women should save it until they're ready for children.

We don't know why some women get endometriosis. To a certain extent it's hereditary, but many other factors seem to come into play. As far as we know, there's nothing you can do to avoid it. It's simply a matter of bad luck. Some grandparents like wintering in Florida while others are happiest staying put, all year round. In the same way, some of us have an endometrium that seems to want to emigrate outside the uterus.

The problem with endometriosis is that there's no sure way of finding out if you have it through simple tests. Blood tests, gynecological examinations, and imaging systems like MRI tell us little or nothing about the charter-hungry endometrium. The only way we can confirm or rule out whether women have endometriosis is to open up their abdomen and look inside. This is done through keyhole surgery—peering into the abdominal cavity with cameras through a small hole. As with all surgery, complications can arise, so this isn't done unless the problems are major and other causes for the pain have been ruled out.

What doctors will often do instead of this surgery is try out endometriosis treatment and see if it works. For most women, the treatment is simple, and harmless, too: contraceptive pills without a break or a hormonal IUD and painkillers, like ibuprofen. By taking contraceptive pills continuously, the endometrium colonies are prevented from bleeding and this can also cause them to shrink over time.[12] Ibuprofen helps with the pain and may reduce inflammation at the same time. This won't eliminate the colonies, but the problems will diminish.

If this kind of treatment doesn't help, there are other more sophisticated ways of treating endometriosis, such as surgery or stronger hormonal treatment. This is specialized work. Unfortunately, the treatment doesn't cure the disease. Even after surgical removal, the endometrium colonies will return over time. Although endometriosis is a chronic disease that doesn't pass until menopause, you should be aware that there is help out there and ways to reduce your pain. The first important step is realizing that it's actually endometriosis you're dealing with and finding a doctor who cares. Awareness of endometriosis is slowly growing, and we sincerely hope we are the last generation of women to grow up without having heard of this potentially disabling disease.

POLYCYSTIC OVARY SYNDROME— WHEN YOUR HORMONES GO HAYWIRE

"The only thing worse than periods is not getting periods," as a female friend of ours likes to say. A lot of women worry if their period vanishes or appears more rarely than once a month. One common cause of irregular menstruation or infrequent menstrual bleeding is a condition called polycystic ovary syndrome, PCOS.

You haven't heard of it before? Well, you're not the only one, but there are good reasons why we should all be more aware of this disease. It is, in fact, the most common hormonal disorder among women of fertile age, affecting somewhere between 4 and 12 percent, many of whom don't know it themselves.[13]

The name of the disease comes from the cysts that are often found on the ovaries with PCOS. These are like small water blisters filled with a transparent fluid, which can make the ovaries look like bunches of grapes. Unlike other types of cysts on the ovaries, these ones are so small that they don't burst, so you won't notice they're there.

Although this is the best-known aspect of PCOS, it's just a small part of the disease. PCOS is a syndrome, meaning that it consists of several different problems that often, although not always, occur together. The problems are caused by a number of hormonal system disorders. They don't just mess with the ovaries, but also the pancreas, the digestive system, and the pituitary gland, that little scrotum-shaped gland in the brain.

The ovaries have the task of storing all your eggs and ensuring that ovulation occurs each month. If you have PCOS, these tasks may become problematic because both the pituitary gland in the brain and the ovaries produce the wrong levels of the hormones that control the menstrual cycle. The result is that you have fewer ovulations or none at all. You'll notice this in your everyday life because your period will arrive more rarely or will disappear entirely.

Since ovulation is necessary in order to become pregnant, many women with PCOS will take longer than normal to conceive, or will need help to do so.[14] PCOS is one of the most common causes of fertility problems among women.[15] It is also linked to a higher risk of complications in pregnancy, such as miscarriage and gestational diabetes.

It is suspected that women with untreated PCOS face a higher risk of endometrial cancer later in life; this is the most common form of genital cancer among women in the Western world.[16] One review study found that while healthy women have a lifetime risk of around three percent of acquiring endometrial cancer, women with untreated PCOS appear to have a risk of 9 percent over their lifetime.[17]

One of the reasons why untreated PCOS is believed to lead to higher risk of endometrial cancer is that the uterine lining of women with PCOS is being built up all the time, but it's not shed through menstruation. As a result, the cells of the uterine lining get "old" and can begin to behave abnormally. This is easily preventable by ensuring that the woman has three or four menstrual bleedings over a year, with the help of contraceptive pills or another course of hormones.

Just to be clear, what's happening with this old uterine lining is not the same thing that happens when people skip their periods using hormonal contraception. With PCOS, the uterine lining is continuously receiving signals telling it to grow, whereas hormonal contraception prevents the lining from growing in the first place. Although the result in both cases is fewer periods, the mechanisms are quite different.

In addition to all the fuss with ovulation, the ovaries—as well as the fatty tissues and the adrenal glands—can produce too much of the male hormones, so-called androgens. All women produce some male sex hormones, but the balance is normally tipped in favor of the female variants. If the androgens get the upper hand, you may find that hair growth increases in places you're not used to having it, such as beard growth on your face or a thick "happy trail"—the broad strip of pubic hair on your stomach. This is called hirsutism and over half of all women with PCOS are troubled by it.[18] A lot of women with PCOS have problems with persistent acne, lasting well beyond puberty. The way they put on weight will also be affected. Women often tend to put on weight in a pear-like pattern—most of the fat settles around their hips and thighs—but with PCOS, male sex hormones mean that women tend to put on weight following an apple pattern—around the belly. You can even end up with a beer gut, one of the most unhealthy types of fat possible. However, androgens also have unnoticeable effects. For example, you may get high levels of cholesterol and fatty acids in the blood, and that's no good for the walls of your blood vessels.

The third area that often behaves abnormally when you have PCOS is the pancreas. This is an organ in the digestive system that produces substances that break down food, as well as a hormone called insulin. Insulin is released after meals and sends the body's cells signals that trigger uptake and consumption of blood sugar. In 50 to 70 percent of women with PCOS, the cells do not react to insulin signals from the pancreas the way they should.[19] These women are insulin resistant and so the pancreas compensates by producing even more insulin, in the hope that the message will finally get through. People aren't laughing at your joke? Talk louder!

This high insulin level isn't good for the body. If you don't get the insulin resistance under control, you may develop type II diabetes over time. Women with PCOS have a much higher chance of developing diabetes than other women with the same weight and lifestyle.[20] American studies have shown that between 20 and 40 percent of PCOS patients are in the preliminary stages of diabetes or have full-blown type II diabetes by the time they reach their forties.[21] The combination of insulin resistance, abnormal levels of fat in the blood, and increased fat around the belly can elevate the risk of cardiovascular disease when you are older.

As you'll have gathered, you should take PCOS seriously. If you have irregular menstruation, polycystic ovary syndrome may be the reason. To check whether you have PCOS, your doctor will measure your hormone levels and examine your ovaries with an ultrasound to check for cysts. If you find you are one of the women out there with PCOS, there are certain things it's important to think about to ensure your future health.

The most vital advice for women with PCOS relates to weight control and lifestyle changes. If you are overweight, you may have fewer problems with PCOS if you lose weight. If your weight is already normal, this won't help. Losing weight can be easier said than done, but any exercise and healthy eating will improve your well-being. In fact, for up to four out of five overweight women with PCOS, losing just 5 percent of their body weight—for example going down from 176 to 167 pounds—is enough to return their normal ovulation.[22] In addition, this can reduce insulin resistance as well as the likelihood of diabetes and cardiovascular disease. The problems with increased hair growth and acne also diminish, because being overweight in itself increases the production of male sex hormones.

We would also advise you to discuss using a combined product, such as contraceptive pills, the contraceptive patch, or the vaginal ring, with a doctor who is knowledgeable about PCOS. This is one of the most important parts of PCOS treatment. The estrogen in contraceptive pills will reduce the production and activity of male sex hormones from the ovaries, which will help with both hair growth and acne. In addition, it's possible to reduce the development of further cysts and the risk of endometrial cancer. Women who cannot take estrogen because of a risk of blood clots can use estrogen-free methods of contraception such as the hormonal IUD or the contraceptive implant, but unfortunately these have no effect on the male hormones.

Think about whether you want children or not. If you do, it may be sensible not to put it off for too long. Many women with PCOS need help to get pregnant and this process takes time. It's a good idea to be prepared for that possibility.

FIBROIDS—A UTERUS WITH BALLS

Did you get an unpleasant surprise last time you were at the gynecologist? A lot of us have benign tumors, known as *fibroids*, in our uterus. Your blood might run cold when you hear the word *tumor* applied to your own body, but in this case you can relax. Just lie back on the gynecologist's table and breathe deeply. Fibroids are benign tumors that grow from cells in the muscle walls of the uterus. They have nothing to do with cancer. They are not cancer now and they will never become cancer. Doctors may refer to fibroids as myomas or "muscle knots," which should make it easier to grasp the difference between benign and slightly less benign tumors.

Fibroids are made of what we call smooth muscle, in other words muscles we cannot control consciously, like the ones we have in our gut and stomach, for example. They are often spherical and rubbery. If you had one on the table in front of you, you could cut it in two with a knife and see that it's actually pearl-white inside, and not red as you might have imagined. Fibroids look a little like pearls—the real ones that grow in oysters at the bottom of the sea.

Fibroids can grow in various places in the uterus—inside the wall, outside the wall, and protruding into the uterine cavity. Some women with fibroids have just one, but it's common for people to have as many as six or seven.[23] They may be tiny or in worse cases they may grow to the size of a grapefruit. Fibroids don't necessarily grow steadily over time. Some may grow an awful lot in a short time, while others will stop when they are one centimeter long, and others still will shrink and vanish of their own accord.

Fibroids are very common among women up to the age of menopause. Like so much else when it comes to the genitals, they respond to estrogen, so they only appear after puberty and tend to vanish after menopause. Up to one in four women discover that they have these myomas.[24] There are probably even more who have them but they're often so small that people don't notice them. Since fibroids are only benign tumors, there's no need to look for them just to check whether they are there or not. It's fine to have them as long as they're not giving you any trouble.

Most myomas involve no symptoms, although you may get severe or prolonged menstrual bleeding, particularly if they are protruding into the uterine cavity. Bleeding between periods is not common, nor is pain a classic sign of myomas, although some women do experience pressure pain in their genitals if their fibroids grow very big. One exception is if a fibroid begins to break up and die, for example owing to poor blood supply. This can be extremely painful and it can be frightening—especially if it happens during pregnancy—but it isn't dangerous.

If you picture the uterus filled with six or seven pearls the size of tennis balls, it's easy to see why fibroids might also cause other problems. They can, for example, press on the bladder, which lies in front of the uterus, giving you a constant urge to urinate. They can also give you a heavy, bloated feeling, slightly reminiscent of pregnancy, and your stomach can, in fact, grow so that it looks as if you're several months along.

In a kind of gruesome irony, the myomas can, in the worst case, make it difficult to get pregnant.[25] Fortunately this applies to a minority of women with fibroids, but they're still the cause of infertility for 1 to 2 percent of women who struggle to have children.[26] It isn't quite certain what prevents pregnancy in women with myomas, but the placement rather than the size seems to be the main cause.[27] Fibroids that protrude into the uterus may make it difficult for the fertilized egg to fasten itself on, because that's precisely where the egg needs to attach itself. The myomas can also block the opening into the fallopian tubes, so that the sperm are unable to reach the egg, which is impatiently waiting for a nice date to fuse with. If fibroids are suspected to be the cause of infertility, they may be removed.[28]

One thing we are more uncertain about is how fibroids affect pregnancy once a woman manages to conceive. Again, it seems to be the myomas that grow into the uterine cavity that cause the most problems. Some studies have shown an increased risk of miscarriage, between 22 and 47 percent, where the fibroids are inward growing.[29] Other than this, fibroids don't seem to have any major adverse effect on the pregnancy, except that Caesarian sections may be done more often if the fibroids are blocking the child's way into the birth canal. So there's usually no reason to surgically remove them before having a baby.[30]

It is possible to limit the growth of fibroids. One simple solution is to try long-acting progestin products such as contraceptives, for example the contraceptive implant or hormonal IUD.[31] If you suffer from heavy bleeding, hormonal contraception can also help combat this. The use of contraceptive methods with a low dosage of estrogen doesn't cause the fibroids to grow, so there's nothing to stop you from using these products if you prefer them.

Generally speaking fibroids in the uterus are a bit like freckles: you may have a few or a lot, big or small, and they don't cause any trouble. There's no need to remove them just because they're there. You only need to remove them if they cause problems. And remember: Fibroids can never become cancer.

VULVODYNIA—UNEXPLAINED PAINS IN THE GENITALS

Are you suffering from pains in your genital area for which neither your doctor nor other health professionals can find an explanation? You are not alone, but the lack of available facts about these pains is frustrating. The pains are there, that's for certain. They take a toll on your everyday life and make it difficult to have sex—but where do they come from? For now, we have little knowledge about this.

All in all, there are many causes of pain in the genital area. Yeast infections and other genital ailments cause persistent burning and itching, and STIs can cause pain during sex. We have painful skin diseases, such as lichen sclerosus, that can affect the vulva and, more rarely, genital cancer can cause pain. Bartholin's glands may become inflamed and extremely painful—the list goes on and on. The thing all these conditions have in common is that they are usually demonstrable. If you see your doctor about the pain, she will examine you and find out the cause of the pain through testing. There's nothing mystifying about genital pain if you have recurring herpes outbreaks, but what if the doctors look and look and can't find anything?

If you have pain in your genital area and cannot find any definite reason for it this is often called vulvodynia. *Dynia* comes from the Greek word for pain. *Vulvodynia* therefore means vulvar pains.[32]

One thing we should emphasize right from the start is that the pains of vulvodynia are absolutely real, even if the doctors can't find any cause for them. Many women with this condition are left feeling as though they're not being taken seriously when they can't get any clear answers about what's wrong with them. Perhaps they've gone through lots of examinations and visited one doctor after another without anybody finding anything wrong at all. Does this mean that the pain is all in their mind? Absolutely not: the pain is real. We do take you seriously.

There are several different ways of having vulvodynia, and this can mean two things: First, that there are several unknown conditions that cause vulvar pain, but since we still know so little about it, we place them under the same umbrella term of vulvodynia. Second, that the different kinds of unexplained vulvar pain may be manifestations of a single condition that produces different symptoms from person to person.

The truth is—along with what causes the pains—we do not know. It will be interesting to see once more research has been done in the field because fortunately medicine is advancing steadily. In the Middle Ages people believed all disease was caused by an imbalance in bodily fluids, and that bloodletting—sometimes with leeches—was a fantastic idea and a miracle cure for everything from depression to cancer. To give you a slightly more recent example, it's not so long since doctors believed stomach ulcers were caused by lifestyle factors such as stress and coffee drinking. However, a particular bacterium called helicobacter pylori turned out to be the culprit.

This may prove to be the case with vulvodynia as well. Is it a neurological disease? A type of bacteria or virus that causes an infection? A reaction to another treatment? We shall see.

Women with vulvodynia may experience different kinds of pain: They may have spontaneous, burning sensations on their genitalia, or what we call *allodynia* and *hyperalgesia* in medical terms. With allodynia, stimuli that don't usually hurt—for example light pressure or touch—suddenly become painful. The touch of a finger can, for example, trigger burning pain on the vulva. Allodynia often occurs in areas of the body that have been injured in some way. We don't know for sure whether this applies to allodynia of the genital area. Hyperalgesia means that stimuli that are usually painful become even more so. For example, a pinprick that you'd normally shrug off can result in intense pain. Both hyperalgesia and allodynia are neuropathic pains. This means that they arise because of an injury to or disease of the peripheral nerves—i.e., the nerves outside the brain and spinal cord.

Burning pains and neuropathic pains are the most common forms of pain associated with vulvodynia, but we can't say for sure that other forms of pain cannot occur. It is possible that the pains themselves vary from person to person and, as mentioned, we don't know whether all instances of vulvodynia are the same disease. Another important factor is that we interpret the pain in different ways. This applies to all pain, not just vulval pain. Some, for example, may experience the discomfort as an itching, and think that it is caused by something they're familiar with from before, such as a yeast infection. This can result in more frequent antifungal treatments even though yeast is not the cause.[33]

There are also variations in where the pain is located, and this is one of the factors that divides vulvodynia into groups. Some people experience pain in their entire vulva—i.e., by the vaginal opening, on the clitoris, and around and on the labia. This is referred to as generalized vulvodynia and is more common among slightly older women. Others have localized pain in a specific place on their vulva. This is called localized vulvodynia and is most common among younger women. It is commonest to experience pains on the clitoris or right beside the vaginal opening, in the area known as the vestibulum, so these two localized vulvodynias each have their own name: clitorodynia and vestibulodynia.

Vulvodynia, and in particular vestibulodynia, were previously known as vestibulitis, a term you may have heard or read about in the media. When a medical term ends in -itis, it means we're talking about an inflammation. Vaginitis, for example, is the same as vaginal inflammation. Since nobody has managed to prove that any inflammation is present in the genitals when women have vulvodynia, doctors have opted to stop using the name vestibulitis. It is more accurate to call it vulvodynia or just vulvar pains.

There is a difference in the way the pains behave. Some women have what is called provoked pain, while others have spontaneous pain. Provoked pain typically involves neuropathic pain, i.e., hyperalgesia or allodynia. Provoked pain means that it hurts when we come in direct contact with the genitals. This can occur in slightly different ways. Touch or pressure that would not normally hurt can cause great pain. Examples could include the pressure of a bicycle saddle, intercourse, tampon use, and direct contact with the clitoris. You can become so sensitive that even the touch of loose-fitting clothes or underwear can cause pain. One test doctors often use to find out whether you're suffering from provoked pain is to press on the painful area with a cotton bud.

Spontaneous pain means that the pain happens suddenly without any contact at all. This is often a burning pain. You may experience a mixture of provoked and spontaneous pain. Some women have a constant burning sensation all the time, while others have pain now and then.[34] Typically, localized vulvodynia most often involves provoked pain, while generalized vulvodynia most often involves spontaneous pain, as well as pains triggered by contact with clothing.[35]

No definite connection has been found between vulvodynia and other genital problems, such as STIs. One popular theory, however, is that there is a connection between vulvodynia and treatment for yeast infections. This doesn't necessarily mean that you'll get vulvodynia from using antifungal treatment. As we wrote earlier, many believe that the vulvar discomfort they experience is caused by yeast infections, and naturally enough, they use antifungal treatment to get rid of the problems. This can make it difficult to decide whether the treatment is causing the problems or the problems result in the treatment.

One study found a relationship between repeated yeast infections and vulvodynia, but the experiment was carried out on mice, so it's difficult to draw any conclusions when it comes to us bipeds.[36] The mice in the study experienced allodynia. The same study also found there was a tendency for the affected area to become extra sensitive. The number of nerve endings capable of perceiving the pain had risen. Based on this study, it may seem as if repeated yeast infections affected the mice's capacity to feel pain from a purely neurological perspective.

Other studies have shown that women with vulvodynia have developed alterations in their genital nerve supply. It may seem as if some women with vulvar pains have grown more pain-sensitive nerve fibers.[37, 38, 39] It is unclear what causes these changes.

GOOD GIRL SYNDROME?

If you've read about vulvodynia in the media, you've probably picked up on the fact that a lot of people focus on the potential psychological aspect of the illness. Many of those treating it, perhaps especially sexologists who deal with the interplay between psyche and sexuality, also highlight this in their work with patients. Might it be that vulvar pain affects women who have sex when they don't actually want to? Could it be that "good girls" are the ones who are affected, or women who've had bad or painful sexual experiences in the past? What about the women who've been exposed to assault or abuse? All these questions have been put forth regarding unexplained vulvar pain. But do they hold up to scrutiny?

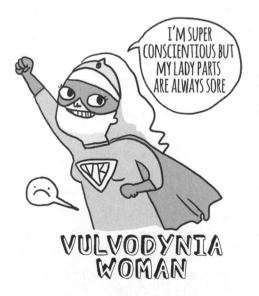

It's easy to slap a "psychological causes" label on conditions whose physical causes aren't immediately identifiable, but we should be very careful about doing this. If women don't recognize themselves in these kinds of descriptions, it can lead to confusion and anger. In particular, the term "good girl" can create a misleading impression that the woman herself, or her personality, is responsible for the pain. This isn't constructive. Genital pains may well turn out to have psychological causes for some women, but that's no cause for shame.

A lot of patients with vulvodynia use talk therapy as part of their treatment. This can have an effect not only because they get to work on potential psychological aspects of the pain, but also because vulvodynia itself can be a major psychological burden that people may need help dealing with.

We know that all kinds of pain are closely linked to the psyche. Many people who experience pain will gradually develop avoidance behavior and tensions that can worsen the underlying problem, leaving the patient trapped in a vicious circle. The expectation that intercourse will be painful can, for example, cause you to unconsciously tense up your vagina to protect yourself, and then the attempts at intercourse will hurt even more.

It is also well known from pain research that the brain becomes more sensitive to new pain impulses when people live with pain over time. Pain simply breeds pain. In both these cases, relaxation techniques and psychotherapy can help people break the cycle. However, this is not the same as claiming that vulvodynia must have a psychological cause from the outset.

As far as we know no research has shown a clear link between vulvodynia and earlier assaults or sexual abuse. Even so, such an experience may be an underlying factor for some women with this condition. Studies that compare the psychological profiles of women with and without vulvodynia yield variable results. One study that compared 240 women with vulvodynia and as many without the condition, showed that it's much more common for vulvodynia to develop among women who have previously suffered anxiety-related conditions.[40] Another study, which compared two smaller groups of women, found no difference in the psychological profiles of women with and without vulvodynia.[41] How far vulvodynia is a disease with a psychological explanation is a matter of debate. It is completely possible to suffer from vulvodynia without having a history of psychological challenges or violent sexual experiences.

Since we know so little about what causes vulvodynia the treatment is still experimental and complex. Different methods that help deal with other pain syndromes are attempted in the hope that they will also help here. Nonetheless the first step is to find a doctor with expertise in the field. There are gynecologists and general practitioners who specialize in vulvar pain.[42]

As we mentioned earlier, neuropathic pains are involved in some forms of vulvodynia and in this case there are some pretty good medicines, for example special antidepressants and some epilepsy medication. These types of medicine, which help combat nerve pain, have proven effective for some women with vulvodynia.[43] Others may find estrogen effective, for example in the form of contraceptive methods such as the vaginal ring. The estrogen affects the mucous membrane in the vagina, making it thicker. Analgesic gel may also reduce the pain, and women struggling with provoked pain who still want to have sex may benefit from this kind of gel during intercourse. In addition to talk therapy, many find physiotherapy helpful. You can learn special exercises that'll make it easier to relax your pelvic floor muscles. Many women with provoked vulvodynia also struggle with other conditions involving muscle tensions, like neck and shoulder pain or tension headaches.

A general piece of advice often given to women with vulvodynia is not to do anything that causes pain. For example, it's important not to force yourself to have intercourse if it hurts. If you want to have sex nonetheless, you can try out other things that don't cause pain, alone or with your partner. Sexologists are good at offering advice and guidance in this respect, and you may want to take your partner, if you have one, to these appointments. People are also advised to be careful about using perfume, soap, and creams on their genitals, as there is some speculation that this may exacerbate the pain.

VAGINISMUS

Many people discuss vulvodynia in the same breath as a condition called vaginismus—which is yet another difficult and somewhat controversial diagnosis. Vaginismus is where a woman involuntarily contracts or has tensions in the pelvic floor muscles that surround the entrance of her vagina. These women often refuse vaginal penetration—whether sexual or for the purpose of a gynecological examination—because they suffer or expect to suffer pain and discomfort. In other words, vaginismus can be a demanding diagnosis, which complicates sex, tampon use, and medical examinations.

Some think of vaginismus as an involuntary muscle spasm that makes the vagina physically narrower. The Norwegian term sometimes used for vaginismus translates as "vaginal cramps." Research using equipment that measures muscle activity has found no clear proof that women with vaginismus have such "muscle spasms," nor is there any professional agreement about which muscles might be involved in vaginismus.[44]

The diagnoses of vestibulodynia and vaginismus overlap. The pains of vaginismus are often described as being the same as or similar to the pains women get with vestibulodynia. The pains are mostly located in the entrance to the vagina and are therefore distinct from the deep pains women get when they have endometriosis or a sore cervix as a result of STIs. Whether these two diagnoses are two sides of the same coin, or two separate conditions that often occur together, is difficult to say.[45]

The treatment for vaginismus is much the same as for vulvodynia. With vaginismus, additional work is often done on training women to be able to tolerate having something in their vagina; this generally starts with the woman herself inserting a very thin object, known as a dilator, whose size is later gradually increased. Analgesic gel is always used during insertion so that it won't be painful.

This element of treatment can be done in collaboration with a gynecologist, sexologist, or physiotherapist.

Vaginismus and vulvodynia are incredibly limiting conditions that take a great toll on women's joie de vivre and sex lives. For many, a normal sex life becomes impossible while the condition persists, and their relationship can deteriorate or fail. Many worry about whether they'll ever have a partner or children, whether they'll have to live alone for the rest of their lives. The fact that we still know so little about these conditions can lead to feelings of bitterness, and many women feel stigmatized in their dealings with their health care providers. One small consolation pending further information is that most women do get better, and many become entirely healthy.

CHLAM, THE CLAP, AND THEIR DISTANT RELATIVES

We're major fans of the *Paradise Hotel* reality TV show, as we mentioned earlier, and we hooted with laughter the time one of the male participants claimed he could tell just by looking at girls whether or not they had venereal disease, and so he never used condoms.[46] We don't know what power he is blessed with. Perhaps he got a certificate from Hogwarts or is related to the Long Island Medium? One thing's for sure, though: nobody can tell just by looking at women (or men) whether or not they have venereal disease. A lot of people don't even know they've been infected themselves—and that's the core of the problem. People keep on having sex without condoms even though they've got venereal diseases. And the thing you don't know about spreads.

We generally call venereal diseases sexually transmitted infections, or STIs for short. STIs can infect you when you have sex or sexual contact with another person who's already been infected. The diseases are caused by different types of microorganisms, such as bacteria, viruses, and parasites. Some of the STIs can only be transmitted through bodily fluids like blood and sperm. Others can be passed on through contact between skin and mucous membranes.

Some STIs are very common, while others are more rare depending on where you live. It's not unlikely that you'll catch one or several STIs in the course of your life. It's one of the few disadvantages of having sex.

Since sexuality has long been associated with shame and guilt—especially for women—the same has also been true of STIs. Even now, few people are open about problems with genital warts and chlamydia. Although these conditions are common and sometimes difficult to protect against, many people are left with the feeling that they should have had less casual sex and avoided exposing their partner to infection. We hope that both knowledge about and normalization of STIs can eliminate some of these awful feelings of shame. Avoiding infection is first and foremost a question of proper condom use and after that, of good and bad luck. It's not a question of your personal sexual morality. Some sleep with hundreds of people without using condoms and miraculously get away without an infection, while others can have a single one-night stand and end up with genital warts. Shit happens in your sexual life, too.

Before we had modern medicine and antibiotics, some STIs were linked to more than just shame. They were also the cause of serious suffering and even death. For a long time, gonorrhea was a common cause of blindness in children, who were infected by their mothers during birth. In the United States, newborns are treated with erythromycin eye ointment shortly after birth for prevention of chlamydia, gonorrhea, and potential E. coli bacterial infections. In Henrik Ibsen's famous 1881 play, *Ghosts*, the suffering artistic soul, Oswald, suffers from syphilis, which ultimately attacks his brain and central nervous system. Today, we can eliminate syphilis with penicillin, enabling people infected with it to return to perfect health. That wasn't possible in 1881, the year *Ghosts* was published. Many people suffered like Oswald and died of the disease.

Despite medical advances, STIs are still a major obstacle to public health worldwide. Since the 1980s, when AIDS began to take the lives of tens of thousands[47] of young gay men, the disease has rarely been out of the news, and with good reason. AIDS, or Acquired

Immune Deficiency Syndrome, is a disease that causes the collapse of the immune defenses—i.e., the body's protection against bacteria and viruses. The microorganism responsible for this is HIV, the human immunodeficiency virus. In 2015, 1.1 million people died of HIV-related causes, and more than 36.7 million people are living with the virus today. Since the start of the epidemic, 35 million people have lost their lives.[48] Once you've been infected with HIV, there's no way to get rid of it. In Norway, HIV-positive people receive such good treatment that they can live a long and almost normal life. With thorough treatment, they will no longer be contagious. There are medicines that can hold the virus in check, but unfortunately, only half of the people in the world who are infected have access to these medicines.

It's a somewhat different story in the United States. While the US does have a good policy on HIV identification, treatment plans, and follow-up, it's individuals with financial means and social status who are best able to manage their disease. In 2014, 37,600 people were infected, a reduction of ten percent from 2010.[49] The CDC estimates that 1.1 million people are living with HIV in the US, but as many as one in seven don't know that they're infected.

The syphilis rate has increased almost every year since 2000–01 in the US. During 2014–15, the national syphilis rate increased 19.0 percent to 7.5 cases per 100,000 population, the highest rate reported since 1994. The rise in the rate of reported syphilis cases is primarily attributable to increased cases among men who have sex with men. However, during 2013–15, the rate increased both among men and women. Men who have sex with men are also the most at risk for contracting HIV, but it's still a good idea for everyone to get tested for HIV at least once along with the regular STI tests that your doctor can perform.

The most common bacterial disease in both the United States and Norway is chlamydia. In 2016, over one and a half million Americans tested positive for chlamydia, and young people under the age of twenty-five are most at risk. The majority of those who test

positive are women: 60 percent of them, no less. This doesn't necessarily mean that women get more chlamydia, but it does mean
they're better at getting themselves tested.

It seems as if some young men choose to rely on women getting
testing, and assume they'll get a phone call if a past partner tests positive. It's not very classy, not to mention being far from watertight as
strategies go. You may well have chlamydia even if your sex partner
has tested negative. The risk of infection isn't 100 percent for every
sexual encounter, and that's why both partners ought to get tested.
In other words, the anti-condom participant in *Paradise Hotel* and
a whole bunch of others along with him really need to change their
habits. Using a condom is always a smart move when you have sex
with a new person, even if you've been tested yourself. There's no
guarantee that your partner will have been as smart as you.

Two illnesses that are a bit like chlamydia are the bacterial diseases mycoplasma and gonorrhea. Gonorrhea is much less common than chlamydia, but still 395,000 cases were reported in the
US in 2015 and rates have been slightly on the rise since reaching
a historic low in 2009. Health professionals are worried about this
rise because of gonorrhea's dramatically increasing antibiotic resistance, making it more important than ever not to get infected in the
first place.

Mycoplasma is a disease that is often overlooked by health professionals. It's a bit like chlamydia's younger sibling. They're very
similar, and have the same symptoms and probably the same
aftereffects—more info about that later. Even so, no routine testing
is done for mycoplasma, unless the patient has symptoms. And even
then, it doesn't occur to many doctors to run tests. The treatment
isn't the same as for chlamydia, so it's important for the disease to
be identified correctly. If you have symptoms but test negative for
chlamydia, it may be sensible to ask for a mycoplasma test.

The most common symptoms of chlamydia, mycoplasma, and
gonorrhea are a change or increase in discharge, a stinging sensation when you urinate, and general discomfort or itching of the
genitals, urethra, or anus, depending on where the infection is

located. The three bacterial diseases often attack the cervix, which becomes inflamed. This can make intercourse unpleasant or painful and some may find they bleed a bit after or during sex due to pressure on the sore cervix. Generally, you should always be alert to any bleeding from the vagina when you don't know what's causing it—particularly if you experience bleeding during or after sex. One explanation may be menstruation or the use of hormonal contraception, for example, but unexplained bleeding may be caused by STIs or other diseases and so it should always be checked by a doctor.

However, not everybody gets symptoms. In fact, only half of all men and as few as a third of all women experience chlamydia symptoms.[50] It's common not to have symptoms with mycoplasma or gonorrhea either, so you might wonder why we should bother about something if we don't even notice it. Well, first off, bacterial diseases are extremely contagious. The risk of infection with chlamydia during unprotected sex is 20 percent.[51] Second, there is a danger of long-term damage.

If the bacteria get the chance, they can find their way up through the cervix and end up in the uterus and the fallopian tubes. There, they can cause inflammation. This is known as pelvic inflammatory disease (PID), and you can get it from chlamydia, mycoplasma,[52*] and gonorrhea. It is estimated that untreated chlamydia will cause 10 to 15 percent of people to develop acute PID.[53] The danger is that the inflammation may cause scarring in the fallopian tubes, blocking them. This is a common reason why women have trouble conceiving, and in addition to infertility it can cause chronic pain. Gonorrhea, in addition to chlamydia, is a major cause of PID for women in the United States.

If you get pelvic inflammatory disease, it is common to feel sick and unwell, and you often experience severe pains in your lower

---

* There is disagreement in professional circles as to how far mycoplasma can cause pelvic inflammatory disease. Research in this field is still sparse, but a few small individual studies suggest this to be the case. Better safe than sorry.

abdomen, vaginal bleeding, fever, and increased discharge. Typically, the pain does not diminish or get better but increases. These types of symptoms should be taken seriously and checked by a doctor as quickly as possible at a women's clinic or urgent care center.

It is also possible, though not common, to have symptom-free PID, which may only be discovered years later during infertility treatment.[54] Voilà: yet another reason to get checked regularly after changing sexual partners.

Chlamydia, mycoplasma, and gonorrhea can be treated with antibiotics. For now, most people who are infected return to full health without long-term damage, but a worrying trend of antibiotic resistance is developing, particularly in the case of mycoplasma and gonorrhea. Antibiotic resistance means that the bacteria become immune to some types of antibiotics, so that more powerful medicines are needed to get rid of them. For this reason, the best option is to avoid getting infected from the outset by using condoms.

There are some STIs that are even more common than chlamydia: herpes and HPV, both of which are viral diseases. HPV is short for human papillomavirus and there are many different forms of the virus. Some types cause genital warts. Others can cause cervical cancer. Herpes is the same as cold sores and is a disease that causes small blisters on the skin.

Herpes and HPV are passed on through contact between skin and mucous membranes. We don't know exactly how many people are infected with the different types, but both are very widespread and it's common for people not to notice that they've been infected.

Because there aren't necessarily any symptoms, many people are infected by a partner who doesn't know that he or she is contagious. This makes it difficult to protect against infection. Nor is it certain that condoms provide good enough protection. If, for example, a man has genital warts or herpes on the root of his penis, he will be able to infect his partner even if he uses a condom. The condom simply doesn't cover the infectious area.

You can be vaccinated against HPV, and some of the vaccines give protection against both the viruses that cause genital warts and those that can cause cervical cancer. If you get genital warts, they can be treated with cryotherapy (frozen with liquid nitrogen) or swabbed with different medications that make them disappear. In other words, it's very much like the treatment you get when you have a plantar wart from the showers at the swimming pool—and in fact, plantar warts are themselves caused by another variant of the human papillomavirus. Genital warts are not dangerous and they have nothing to do with the risk of cancer. Warts and cancer are tied to different types of HPV.

HPV infections will often pass of their own accord. The warts will, too, but some people's warts continue to come back.

Herpes, meanwhile, is a virus you cannot get rid of. Once you've been infected, the virus will remain in your nerve cells in a kind of hibernation for the rest of your life. You may have several outbreaks, which can be shortened with a course of prescription pills. However, herpes isn't dangerous and the symptoms tend to diminish over time.

HOW CAN I PROTECT MYSELF AGAINST STIs?

Condoms provide good protection against HIV, chlamydia, mycoplasma, and gonorrhea. However, HPV and herpes can be passed on through skin contact, so you can be infected from places that are not covered by the condom.

When performing oral sex on a woman, you can use a dental dam—a thin, transparent sheet of latex that can be placed over the vulva. This will, for example, be able to prevent herpes infection from mouth to genitals or from genitals to mouth. Dams are available for purchase online or in sex toy shops. You can also make your own by snipping the top off a condom, cutting the length of the cylinder, and spreading it out so that you get a large, transparent square.

WHEN SHOULD I GET TESTED?

It's sensible to get tested for chlamydia every time you have unprotected sex with a new partner, even if you don't have any symptoms. It's also a good idea for you and your partner to get checked as early in your relationship as possible. Since you can have venereal diseases for a long time without noticing anything wrong, you may in fact both have chlamydia without knowing it.

If you've had unprotected anal sex, it isn't certain that the infection will be picked up if you don't also take a test anally. In that case, you should ask for an anal test.

If you have symptoms of any kind, you should have a genital examination. It's important to contact your doctor if it stings when you urinate, if you have itching, if your discharge changes, if you have a rash, blisters, or unusual bleeding, or if there are any other things you notice that are out of the ordinary.

It is important to be aware that a chlamydia test is only deemed effective if it is taken at least two weeks after you were potentially exposed to infection. Many people test positive before the two weeks are up, and that's fine, because it means that treatment can begin earlier. If you get a positive result before two weeks have passed, you can be sure that you have chlamydia—but if the result of an early test is negative, you can't be entirely certain of it until you take a new test, at earliest two weeks after the sex in question. What we're saying is, early testing will not result in false positives for chlamydia, but there can be false negatives in the first two weeks after contracting the disease. This two-week rule also applies to testing for mycoplasma and gonorrhea.[55] In other words, there is no reason to panic and schedule an appointment with your gynecologist first thing Monday morning after a raucous weekend.

RISK AND DANGEROUS VACATION SEX

We've discussed a long list of venereal diseases but focused on the chlamydia test. What about the other diseases? Some women go to the doctor and ask to be tested for "everything," but there's no need to get tested for everything every time. Which tests you should take is something you should decide with your doctor, and this will depend on what risk you've had of becoming infected with a venereal disease.

Among young women in the United States, chlamydia is absolutely the most common venereal disease and it's often enough to test for that. Your risk of serious diseases such as HIV and syphilis is relatively low, unless you engage in so-called high-risk sex.

However, if you've had unprotected sex while you've been on vacation abroad, it's important to tell your doctor. Doctors often forget to ask, so don't expect them to take the initiative. The same applies if you've had sex with somebody who's just returned from traveling in a country with a lot of venereal diseases. And just to set the record straight, it's worth being aware that this also applies to countries that have very good reputations for medical care—they might still have quite different incidences of venereal disease.

If you've sold or bought sex, you should definitely take a broader range of tests. The same applies if you've injected drugs or have had sex with a person who does so.

In Norway and the United States,[56] the group consisting of men who have sex with men (MSM) has the highest risk of contracting more serious venereal diseases.* Gonorrhea and syphilis are much more common among MSM than in the heterosexual population. This makes it extra important for these men to get tested. It may be good to remember that this also applies to women who have sex with MSM. If your last male one-night stand also has sex with men, your risk of disease is higher too. The focus on MSM isn't about shaming people—it's a question of statistics, and of looking after your health.

You may have good or bad luck whether you have sex with women, men, or men who have sex with men. It won't do any harm

---

* We use the term "men who have sex with men" in preference to "homosexual." It is quite possible to be a man who has sex with men without identifying as homosexual. Sexual orientation is not necessarily the same as who you have sex with.

to test yourself for less common diseases, but if the risk isn't especially high, you don't need to do it every time you have a sexual encounter. Test often, test according to the risk, and use condoms as often as possible.

HERPES—IS YOUR SEX LIFE OVER?

Small, painful blisters on your lips or your genitals aren't fun, but nonetheless, herpes is more common than you think. It's infectious, a nuisance, and impossible to protect against, but fortunately it's harmless. Even so, it seems as if herpes is the venereal disease a lot of people are most frightened of.

Many are scared by the fact that you can't get rid of herpes. Once you've been infected, the virus will be in your body for the rest of your life. This raises a lot of questions. Does it mean, for example, that you're always infectious and that you can never have sex with anybody without a condom again?

The sudden appearance of herpes in a relationship also creates a lot of distrust and uncertainty. Who infected whom? Has your partner of three years been unfaithful to you?

There are a lot of myths and misunderstandings about herpes. Anxiety about herpes is common, both among those who are infected and those who are afraid of infection.

Herpes is a viral disease that affects the skin and mucous membranes. Two slightly different viruses may be the culprits: herpes simplex virus 1 (HSV-1) and herpes simplex virus 2 (HSV-2). The herpes virus is transmitted through contact with the skin or mucous membrane, such as through kissing or sex. It can also be transmitted indirectly. The classic example is the kindergartner who is infected after sucking on the same plastic dinosaur as other children. Over half of the population is probably infected with HSV-1 on their mouth during childhood.[57]

According to the Centers for Disease Control and Prevention, approximately one out of six people in the United States aged fourteen to forty-nine has genital herpes caused by HSV-2. Worldwide

rates of either HSV-1 or HSV-2 are estimated to be between 60 percent and 95 percent in adults.[58] For once it's almost correct to say
that *everybody* has it, unlike that time you tried to convince your
dad that *everybody else* had a Game Boy and that you had to have
one, too. You may be infected with both types or just one of them.
On top of that, it's possible that an even larger share of the population has herpes. A lot of those who are infected don't know a thing
about it, because not everybody gets the associated symptoms.

Just stop and think about these figures a bit. This means that it's
more common to be infected with herpes than not. Even so, a lot of
people think of herpes as being the end of the world. But more than
60 percent of the world population haven't had their lives destroyed
or found themselves unable to have sex again!

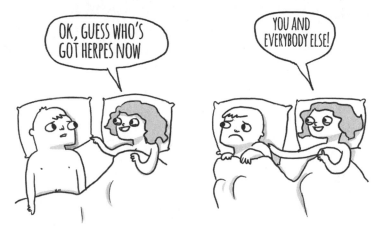

But hang on a second. Oral herpes and genital herpes are two different diseases, aren't they? So why are we talking about them as if
they were the same thing? A sexually transmitted infection is pretty
different from a cold sore, isn't it?

Herpes is, in fact, the same wherever you have it on your body.
Before, it was thought that HSV-1 was mostly linked to oral herpes, and HSV-2 to genital herpes. But HSV-1 can just as easily cause
outbreaks on the genitals and HSV-2 can just as easily cause an outbreak on the lips, assuming that this is where you've been infected.
You can also get herpes around the anus, on your fingers, or (if

you're really unfortunate) in your eye. That said, HSV-1 on the genitals involves fewer and milder symptoms than HSV-2.[59]

It's possible to transmit the infection from genitals to lips and even more common the other way. Most young women who contract genital herpes these days are actually infected by HSV-1 from the lips of a partner during oral sex. This applies to as many as 80 percent.[60]

Since so many people have herpes without knowing about it, this means in practice that many young women are infected by a partner who doesn't know that he or she has herpes. So how are you supposed to protect yourself against it?

Once you've been infected, the virus can cause an outbreak within a couple of days, but it is also possible to be infected without noticing anything. After infection, a gang of herpes viruses will move up the nerves from the area of skin where the infection occurred. They'll settle down to sleep inside a nerve cell a bit deeper in your body, like a bear going into hibernation. And there they will remain for the rest of your life. Now and again, the virus will move down through the nerves and out onto your skin, and then a new outbreak may occur, causing blisters to form in the same place as last time. It is also possible to have a "hidden outbreak"—i.e., the virus may be on the skin without you noticing anything at all.

A visible herpes outbreak starts with discomfort in the form of a prickling, burning sensation on the skin of your genitals or your lips. Then small blisters appear, growing in clusters, several crowded together. After a few days, the blisters dry out and become scabs, which eventually fall off.

The first outbreak is usually the worst. It is known as a primary herpes outbreak and can make some people very ill. They may have a fever or problems urinating because the stinging in their genitals is so bad. As with everything else, you should visit your doctor if you get severe symptoms without knowing for sure what the problem is. A primary herpes outbreak will last longer than later outbreaks. You may get new blisters for one to two weeks. The scabs will disappear entirely three or four weeks after that.[61] If you have a

dramatic primary outbreak, it may help to think that the next outbreak won't be as bad—if indeed you have another outbreak at all.
Many people never have any more after the first one.

If you do have a new outbreak, it will always happen in the same
place where you were first infected. The number of outbreaks will
usually diminish over the years. There is no medicine that can get
rid of the herpes, but there is a course of pills you can take to calm
and shorten the outbreak if you notice that it's imminent. In especially troublesome cases involving many outbreaks each year, you
can use medication over longer periods to suppress outbreaks.

New outbreaks often come at times when your immune defenses
are low. That's why the common name for oral herpes is cold sore.
You often get it when you're ill, for example with a cold. Stress, menstruation, or sun can also trigger an outbreak, as can irritation of
the skin—for example, chafing underwear and waxing or shaving.

There is no vaccine against herpes, as there is with the HPV virus,
but there's actually no need for one. Herpes acts a bit like a vaccine
against itself: If you've been infected with it once, for example as a
child, you can't be infected with the same virus on another place on
your body later in life. The virus activates your immune defenses
so that they'll always recognize the same virus and prevent it from
settling in new nerve cells. That means you'll only be infected in
one place by each virus. If you're infected on the mouth, you're protected against infection of the genitals and vice versa—and for the
same reason, you can't infect yourself in other places if you have an
outbreak in one spot. Watch out, though! That only applies once
the immune system has been activated. Your immune defenses take
a bit of time to build up to recognizing herpes, so you can, in fact,
spread your infection the first time you have an outbreak with one
of the herpes types. You should be extra careful about hand washing and hygiene if you're having an outbreak for the first time. Don't
rub your eyes when you've got virus on your fingers. Just don't do it!

To complicate matters, as you now know, there are two herpes
viruses. If you've previously been infected with HSV-1, you won't
be protected against infection by HSV-2. In theory, you can get

herpes in two places if the two different herpes viruses are involved. However, you have a certain degree of cross-protection. If you're infected with a second virus, you often get milder symptoms or no symptoms at all.[62]

Even though you can't infect yourself once the first outbreak is over, you *can* infect others. The most common question we get about herpes is: When am I contagious? Naturally enough, people with genital herpes are scared of infecting others—and how are you supposed to know you're safe? Can treatment with medication prevent infection, or are there special times when you shouldn't have sex?

For transmission to occur through skin and mucous membrane contact, the virus must be on the skin or the mucous membranes. Since herpes usually lies hibernating in the nerve cells deep in the body, you're not usually contagious. The virus must have moved out from the nerves and onto the skin in order for you to be able to infect other people. This is something that happens when you have an outbreak. You are most contagious a week before an outbreak, because that's when the virus is gathering on the skin, as well as during the outbreak itself. The blisters are full of the virus. It may be sensible to avoid sex when you feel that an outbreak is on the way—which often happens several days before the blisters appear. Of course, it can be difficult to know for certain that an outbreak is imminent a week before it arrives.

And then there are the hidden outbreaks, too. The virus can wander out onto the skin, making you contagious, without you noticing anything at all and without you getting any blisters. In practice that means that you *can* be contagious at any time. You can never be certain that you're not contagious. There are no safe periods. By now you may be thinking: *But that's a total crisis!* It's quite simply impossible to be certain that you won't infect other people, and that's probably the most difficult aspect of being infected. But don't lose hope.

Let's say that you have HSV-1 of the genitals and want to have sex with a new person. There's a 70 percent chance that your potential partner has already been infected with the virus and is therefore protected against new infection without knowing it. That alone reduces the risk dramatically. If, in addition, your partner has a cold sore on her mouth, you can be almost certain that you won't infect her, since oral herpes is usually caused by HSV-1.

Another way of looking at it is that most people will be infected sooner or later regardless. If you don't infect them, somebody else will at a later time. Herpes is harmless and most of the people who have the virus hardly notice.

Finally, we need to talk about a difficult problem connected with herpes: herpes in a relationship. Let's say that neither you nor your partner has had herpes blisters before. Not on your mouths, not on your genitals. You've been together for three years and have a fantastic relationship. And then it happens. You get a severe outbreak of blisters on your genitals and think the worst. You haven't been with anybody else, so your partner must have, right?

As you now know, you won't necessarily be aware that you have herpes. It's not a given that you had an outbreak of blisters when you were infected. You may have had herpes for a long time without having a visible outbreak. It's also quite possible you've been infected by one of your partner's invisible outbreaks. In other words, infidelity need not have come into the picture at all. Herpes is common and you don't necessarily know you have it. We've seen relationships ruined by unfounded accusations of infidelity after a herpes outbreak. Of course, it's possible infidelity may have been involved, but herpes is no proof of that. If you don't have any other reason to doubt your partner, herpes shouldn't be the factor that sows the seeds of distrust.

It's great for people to take responsibility for not infecting their partners with venereal diseases. If we were talking about chlamydia, we'd applaud loudly, but when it comes to herpes, it often just makes us sad. It's so unnecessary for people to be afraid of having sex because of herpes. Herpes isn't HIV, even though both are viruses you can't get rid of. Herpes is ultimately harmless. It isn't the end of the world to be infected with genital herpes. You're one of many—in fact, one of the majority. It's highly likely it will give you very few problems over the course of your life. And if you do have symptoms, the chances are that they'll diminish. If you do have lots of outbreaks, treatment is available, including a medication called Valtrex that lessens the symptoms of an outbreak.

INTENSE ITCHING AND ROTTEN FISH— GENITAL PROBLEMS YOU'LL CERTAINLY ENCOUNTER

Something's brewing between your legs. It's red and it smells peculiar, or it's itching so much you can't sleep at night. Yeast infections and bacterial vaginosis are common genital problems that aren't caused by sexually transmitted infections. Most women are hit by one or the other, or both, over the course of their lives. Both conditions are harmless, but they can be an incredible nuisance. Since you'll probably encounter these genital problems, it may be worth finding out a bit more about them.

Microorganisms such as bacteria and fungus usually trigger negative associations and a yearning for soap and disinfecting wipes. Who hasn't heard how quickly bacteria can multiply on a dishcloth, or seen how fungus spreads across a wall in a damp cellar? It's enough to give you the shudders—but not all microorganisms are harmful.

Some bacteria are totally necessary for us to function, such as the gut bacteria that assist our digestion. In fact, we have around ten times as many bacteria as we have cells in our bodies, and that doesn't mean that we are ill.

The mucous membrane on the vulva and in the vagina is covered with microorganisms that constitute what is known as the normal flora of the genitals. The normal flora helps keep your vagina healthy by supporting the immune system in its battle against alien microorganisms and by keeping the vaginal environment in balance. As you may remember, the vagina is self-cleaning, and the use of soap and, especially, douches eliminates the natural protection of the genitals—partly because it wipes out the normal flora.

The vagina's normal flora varies according to your current life stage. Before you enter puberty and after menopause, the normal flora consists mostly of skin and gut bacteria, but when you're fertile, your body is influenced by estrogen. This makes the mucous membrane thick and active, and the normal flora becomes unique to your genitals. It differs from the normal flora in other parts of your body.

The normal flora of fertile women consists for the most part of different types of lactic acid bacteria, called lactobacilli, which rely on estrogen for their nourishment and survival. The lactobacilli produce acid like the type you find in yogurt. Lactic acid ensures that the vagina has a low pH of around 4.5. This creates an environment that is inhospitable to bad bacteria types, which aren't comfortable in acidic surroundings. In addition, there are a couple of other bacteria types: some yeast fungus and some virus.[63] All the microorganisms are battling for the same food and a place to live, and since there are so many different types, none of them will gain the upper hand. Together with the body's immune defenses, the different microorganisms keep one another in check. The genitals are vulnerable to problems when the protective normal flora becomes imbalanced.

YEAST INFECTIONS IN THE VAGINA

Let's start off with yeast infections. Around 20 percent of all women have a kind of yeast known as Candida albicans as part of their vagina's normal flora.[64] Many have this kind of yeast in their butt and it may move from there to the vagina, especially if the opportunities for growth there are good. As many as 50 percent of all pregnant women have yeast in their vaginas.[65] This may be because Candida albicans loves estrogen and the body is extra full of estrogen when you're pregnant. Candida albicans is responsible for the vast majority of yeast infections in the United States.

Hang on, though. *Yeast*—you mean the stuff that makes rolls and bread light and fluffy? Almost! It isn't exactly the same type of yeast you find at the supermarket, but it's similar. In fact, one woman with a yeast infection used yeast from her vagina to produce sourdough in November 2015 and became a genuine Internet sensation in the process.[66] Her method was to collect a bit of her discharge using a dildo. The sourdough worked and she baked a loaf, which she then ate. She said it tasted "pretty damn nice."

If you're among the 20 percent whose vagina always contains yeast, this doesn't mean you have a yeast infection; that only happens when the yeast causes inflammation of the mucous membrane. In other words, when you've got it, you'll know it.

This yeast infection can affect both the interior of the vagina and the inner labia. The itching may be intense, and some women also find that it stings or burns down below. This can make intercourse painful or cause a stinging sensation in your vulva when you urinate. The infected mucous membrane becomes red and swollen. Some women also get a whitish, lumpy discharge that can be described as looking like cottage cheese, while others get a runny discharge.

Some women find that when they have a yeast infection in their vagina, their male partners develop symptoms on their penis, such as a rash or an itching sensation. Nonetheless, we must stress that a yeast infection is not a sexually transmitted infection. You can still have sex while you're being treated for one if it doesn't cause you pain, but you might want to hold off until your symptoms are in check because the inflammation you experience can be further irritated by intercourse. If a male partner gets a rash, they don't usually need separate treatment—but if you find that you're having recurring yeast infections, you could be passing the fungus back and forth.

Since yeast infections are so common, treatment is sold over the counter at the drugstore. There are many types and all of them work pretty well. The treatment consists of a cream and vaginal suppositories, or antifungal pills you take orally. If you use the vaginal suppository, you should insert it before you go to bed so that it can do its work overnight. If not, the suppository has a tendency to dissolve and rapidly run out into your underwear. If you use the cream, you need to smear a thin layer of it on your inner labia, all the way from your clitoris to your anus. It may be a good idea to avoid vaginal suppositories when you're having your period, not because it's harmful but because the blood can carry the medication out of the vagina—flush it out, so to speak.

The availability of these over-the-counter treatments lowers the threshold for women to diagnose and treat themselves when they have the symptoms of a yeast infection.

The problem there is that *all that itches is not yeast*! If it itches down below, there's only a 50 percent likelihood that it's a yeast infection.[67] Different genital conditions can resemble one another. So we recommend in the strongest possible terms that women who suffer new symptoms should visit their doctor. Itching and changes in discharge are vague symptoms that can have many different causes, e.g., sexually transmitted infections such as chlamydia and gonorrhea, and it's worth identifying problems like that as early as possible. Different types of eczema and irritating conditions of the genitals are also common, sometimes due to residual detergent in your underwear or the use of perfumed soaps or intimate wipes.

It turns out that women are bad at distinguishing between yeast infections and other genital conditions, even if they've had a yeast infection before. Women only diagnose yeast infections correctly in one out of three cases.[68] If, in all these cases, they opt for over-the-counter treatment instead of a trip to the doctor, this leads to a lot of pointless, incorrect treatment that doesn't help eliminate the real problem. Unnecessary use of antifungal treatments can also delay discovery of the actual illness, causing new, additional symptoms. In fact, extensive use of antifungal medication can itself cause an irritation of the mucous membrane that is reminiscent of a yeast infection. In other words, there's nothing stupid about taking a trip to the doctor to make sure it really is a yeast infection—at least the first time you have problems or if you find that the symptoms are constantly recurring.

When you've been diagnosed with a yeast infection and use anti-fungal medication, it's important to use the treatment the way your doctor or pharmacist recommends. Even if the problems go away, you must always complete the course. Continue to use the cream for at least two days after the symptoms disappear, otherwise the infection can easily come back again. If you finish the treatment too early, there's a risk that small amounts of yeast will remain, and then the infection may blow up again when you stop.

Yeast infections are common. We know that three out of four women get them over the course of their lives. But what causes them? It's not so easy to put a finger on it. We know of several things that predispose us to yeast infections. We know that many women get them after using antibiotics, or because they wash their genitals too often. After all, soap and antibiotics will help eliminate the normal flora that keeps our genitals healthy. We also know that estrogen has something to do with it. Prepubescent and postmenopausal women rarely have problems with yeast since their genitals are not as influenced by sex hormones, whereas pregnant women can be troubled by it frequently. We know yeast infections often appear at particular points in the menstrual cycle. Women most often get them before menstruation.

Diabetics are especially prone to them, particularly those with poor control of their blood sugar. We also see that girls get yeast infections more often once they've become sexually active, and those who have sex several times a month are somewhat more predisposed to it.

Some women have long-term problems with yeast infections that never entirely go away. It can be a great hindrance for these women. Three to five percent of all women get more than four yeast infections a year.[69] If you're very prone to it, it's important to talk to your doctor to get a full examination, and to consider antifungal treatment that is stronger than the over-the-counter products.

Unfortunately, no effective method of protecting against yeast infections has been found. However, folk remedies are rife, both on the Internet and at the doctor's office. One common piece of advice is to supplement the lactic acid bacteria in your vagina with yogurt, either in pill form or by drinking lots of probiotic yogurt drinks such as DanActive. However, this kind of treatment hasn't been proven to be effective, so it might be a waste of money, unless you're very fond of DanActive.[70]

Other than that, people are generally advised to keep their genital area dry, as yeast likes wet, warm conditions. This means that you should avoid synthetic underwear and tight pants and jeans, and only use panty liners when strictly necessary. Wear cotton underwear because it breathes best and sleep naked or without underwear or pajama bottoms so that your genitals aren't constricted. None of this has any documented scientific effect, but it may be worth trying if you're really bothered by yeast infections. After all, sleeping in the buff is free and has no dangerous side effects.

BACTERIAL VAGINOSIS

Another genital condition that's also incredibly common is bacterial vaginosis, or BV for short. Have you ever heard female genitals described in fish-related terms—as a shrimp fest or a fish taco? The truth is that healthy genitals shouldn't smell fishy, but BV is to blame for the fact that many do smell that way.

BV is caused by an imbalance of the genitals' normal flora. There is a reduction in the protective lactic acid bacteria, while the other types of bacteria that cause trouble in the environment flourish. The lactic acid bacteria keep your vagina acidic, and acidic is good. When you have BV, your vagina becomes a little less acidic, i.e., more alkaline. That's why pH is one of the things your doctor may measure when you have genital problems to check whether you have BV.

There isn't any one type of bacteria that's solely responsible for BV: it's a cocktail of different kinds. Some of the bacteria usually live in the vagina or in other areas of the body as part of your normal flora. The problem is that they have moved, or that there are too many of them.

Most experts believe that only women who have had sex get BV, and that the risk of acquiring it increases with the number of sexual partners and diminishes with condom use. This applies to both women who have sex with women and women who have sex with men. The more partners, the more BV.[71] So you might think some of the bacteria come from your sexual partner, but that doesn't mean BV is considered to be a sexually transmitted infection. Remember that many different bacteria cause BV. It's not a question of one contagious and harmful bacteria, as with chlamydia. It makes more sense to think of it in terms of mixing up your normal flora with those of several people who have a slightly different combination of bacteria than you. Too many cooks spoil the broth, or in this case spoil the balance.

Women who haven't had several sexual partners may also get BV, but they must still have had sex. BV is considered to be harmless, so there's no reason to protect a regular partner against infection by using a condom or abstaining from sex while you're being treated. It's always worth using a condom if you have several partners, but that's because of the risk of catching sexually transmitted infections, not BV.

In addition to the characteristic smell, which is described as "rotten fish," women with BV have heavier-than-normal discharge. Many describe a grayish, very runny discharge and need to change their underwear several times a day. The smell can be so strong that it can be detected through clothing.

Many women experience a sporadic fishy smell or a worsening of the fishy smell after vaginal intercourse or during and after menstruation. Does that mean that menstruation and sex give you BV? No, but menstruation and sperm can worsen the symptoms if you have BV.

In fact, the smell becomes stronger the more alkaline your genitals become. This means that it becomes worse if you have fewer lactic acid bacteria or if an alkaline substance is added to your vagina. Both blood and sperm are more alkaline than the environment in the vagina and will therefore increase the fishy smell. If you get a fishy smell after your period or after sex it may mean that you have BV without severe symptoms, which flares up when the environment becomes less acidic.

Perhaps this sounds pretty easy to recognize, but as with yeast infections, you won't necessarily recognize BV by its symptoms. Women with BV often get itching and other symptoms that may remind them of a yeast infection. Discharge is a common symptom of different sexually transmitted infections, and it's always possible to have several things at once! It's difficult to distinguish genital conditions from one other. The moral is that you must visit your doctor for a checkup if your genitals are different than normal. Change in discharge, itching, or a stinging sensation? Just go to the doctor.

Bacterial vaginosis doesn't mean that your genitals are dirty, although that's what a lot of people think when they detect the bad smell. If you try to get rid of the problem by washing, you'll only make matters worse by flushing out the good bacteria that keep your vagina acidic. BV can pass of its own accord, but it's best to get medical treatment. Since BV is caused by bacteria, antibiotics or antibacterial treatments are called for. Vaginal suppositories containing lactic acid bacteria are also sold for BV, which supposedly help the environment in the vagina. Unfortunately, there is no research proving that this kind of treatment has any effect whatsoever.

WHEN PEEING HURTS

It's no coincidence that urinary tract infections are sometimes described as "peeing barbed wire." Urinary tract infections are awful and as a woman you're particularly prone to them.

Our short urethra is to blame, and the fact that our anus is in close quarters to the urethral opening. Bacteria from our butt work best if they stay where they belong, but it's difficult to fence them in. They can easily climb into the urethral opening and move up through it until they have settled on the mucous membranes inside the urethra and bladder. Once there, they cause inflammation.

You'll notice a urinary tract infection because it hurts when you urinate. It stings, burns, and can feel as if what's coming out is jagged. It becomes particularly painful toward the end of the flow, when the bladder is emptying itself out entirely and its walls press against each other. In addition, you'll notice that you have a frequent urge to urinate but will only pee a little at a time. You may notice that your urine smells different, or that there's some blood in it.

The vast majority of urinary tract infections in young women—as many as 95 percent—are what we call uncomplicated.[72] This means that the infection is considered to be less dangerous and requires more simple treatment because the bacterial invasion has occurred in a structurally and functionally normal urinary tract.[73] Nonetheless, antibiotics are almost always prescribed in the United States to treat urinary tract infections. Doctors also recommend drinking plenty of water to flush bacteria from the bladder. Anytime you're prescribed antibiotics, it's important to finish the entire course you've been instructed to take, even if your symptoms have disappeared, to ensure that the infection doesn't gain resistance to the antibiotic without being fully eradicated from your body.

Of course, you should always be alert to any worsening of symptoms. If you get a fever or more severe pain, especially if it moves up toward your back, you must visit your doctor as soon as possible or visit an urgent care center. This may be a sign that the bacteria have caused pyelonephritis, which can seriously damage your kidneys.

A urinary tract infection must always be taken seriously if you're pregnant. In that case it is automatically considered to be complicated and you need a special antibiotic treatment. It is also considered to be complicated if you have frequent urinary tract infections. In those cases it's often necessary to investigate more closely what kind of bacteria are involved, and sometimes tests will be carried out to see if you have an underlying condition that makes it easier for you to become infected. Having said that, some women inexplicably get urinary tract infections again and again. It's suspected that these women may have slightly different immune defenses in the mucous membranes of their urinary tract that make it easier for the bacteria to gain a foothold.

Many women desperately seek ways to avoid urinary tract infections. Cranberry juice or pills are common folk remedies that have been used for centuries. Cranberry contains a substance that is supposed to prevent bacteria from attaching themselves to the mucous membrane in the bladder. However, a major review of the research by the prestigious Cochrane Library indicates that cranberry has no protective effect.[74] But again: If you like cranberry juice there's nothing to stop you trying it. Cranberry juice has no side effects. Other tips are to drink large quantities of water to flush out your plumbing, empty your bladder as soon as you need to urinate, and, of course, always wipe from front to back after emptying your bowels.

We do know that sex increases the chances of getting a urinary tract infection. During sex a lot of moisture often builds up in the genitals, making it easier for the bacteria to move from place to place, and at the same time all that genital-to-genital rubbing and thrusting can push bacteria into the wrong hole. The risk of getting a urinary tract infection is sixty times as high as normal in the first two days after intercourse for women under the age of thirty.[75]

You've probably heard the popular advice that if you urinate after sex you'll have a lower chance of ending up with bothersome stinging. It's great advice. By peeing after sex, you'll flush out any gut bacteria that have found their way up into the urethra, getting rid of them before they manage to invade your mucous membrane and cause trouble.

An ordinary urinary tract infection is not a sexually transmitted infection even though sex may be involved—it's just a matter of regular butt bacteria in the wrong place. But chlamydia, gonorrhea, and mycoplasma are also common causes of a stinging sensation when urinating. As such, you should be on the alert. However, the sexually transmitted bacteria behave slightly differently. They thrive in the urethra but not in the bladder, unlike the butt bacteria. When you have a sexually transmitted infection you don't get the characteristic pain at the end of flow. It's also less common to have a frequent urge to urinate. Even so it isn't easy to notice the difference yourself. A urinary tract infection can resemble chlamydia and chlamydia can resemble a urinary tract infection—don't hate us, but it's even possible to get both at once. For this reason, it's always recommended to go to the doctor when you experience symptoms that you think could be a UTI—people often identify infections incorrectly, so it's better to be safe and make sure you're getting the correct treatment.

DRIP, DRIP, DRIP—ALL ABOUT URINE LEAKS

It's no fun having to buy Depends undergarments when you're nineteen and childless, but old ladies and women who have given birth a few times aren't the only ones who suffer from urine leaks. The technical term for leakage is urinary incontinence and it's a widespread problem among women.

Age and childbirth, along with high body mass index (BMI), are the biggest risk factors for urine leaks, which means that an ever-increasing number of women start to suffer from them as they age. That's probably also the reason why many people believe it's uncommon to have urine leaks before giving birth, but women of all ages can be affected.

It's difficult to say just how many women actually suffer from urine leaks. The figures from studies vary and it's believed that fewer than half of all women who have incontinence go to the doctor, which may indicate that the numbers we have are vastly underestimated.[76] One study of Norwegian women found that 30 percent suffered urine leaks,[77] while a study of women three months after giving birth found that 20 to 30 percent were affected.[78] Some international studies have reported anything from 10 to 60 percent, depending on the severity of the leaks involved.[79]

We know less about younger, childless women, and the figures that do exist vary dramatically. One study looking at Australian women between sixteen and thirty who hadn't had children found that as many as 12.6 percent experienced urine leaks.[80] A Swedish study resulted in quite different findings: Around 3 percent of all women aged twenty to twenty-nine had urine leaks.[81]

Regardless of which of these studies comes closest to the truth, we can safely say that urine leaks aren't uncommon among young, childless women.

There are several ways of being incontinent. We distinguish between what is called stress incontinence, urge incontinence, and a mixed form that combines the two.

Stress incontinence is the most common, affecting around 50 percent of those who suffer urine leaks.[82] Stress incontinence is where you leak urine when something causes the pressure on your abdomen to increase, for example when you cough or sneeze, laugh, jump, run, or engage in similar activity. By comparison with urge incontinence, the amounts involved are small, but the degree of severity varies enormously. There may be a difference between how often you leak and how much you leak once it happens.

Urge incontinence is about *need*. Women who suffer from this form of incontinence have a sudden, strong need to urinate right NOW, followed by a large urine leakage. Of all women who have incontinence, 10 to 15 percent have only this form.[83] Women with urge incontinence often have an overactive bladder and that means they have a strong urge to urinate without necessarily leaking. Women with overactive bladders usually pee more often than other women and often have to get up to go in the middle of the night.[84]

Between 35 and 50 percent of women with incontinence have a mixed form, i.e., both stress and urge incontinence. In other words, the form of the leakage can vary. Sometimes you leak when you jump or sneeze, other times you have a powerful urge to urinate and leak a large amount.

Urine leakage can be caused by many things. If you drink more water than you need to, it may be a good idea to cut down. Many people think drinking a lot of water is healthy in itself, but you don't need more than around a half gallon every twenty-four hours unless you exercise a lot or live in an extremely hot climate. You get some of this water through food. It may also be a good idea to cut down on diuretic drinks such as coffee and tea.

Urine leaks may be symptomatic of other illnesses. Some women have leakages when they have a urinary tract infection and some neurological diseases can cause leaks. It may be sensible to discuss urine leaks with your doctor if you can't see any clear reason why they've started, for example that you began to leak after giving birth or after you suddenly began drinking a gallon of water a day. Your doctor can give you guidance and help find a solution.

The fact that you leak urine doesn't necessarily mean you're condemned to wear black clothes on your bottom half to hide the wet spots, or to give up running and laughing for the rest of your life. Fortunately, you can do something about it. The first thing people try requires a bit of initiative. A lot of people who suffer from stress incontinence do so because their pelvic floor muscles are too weak—they may, for example, have been affected after birth. The pelvic floor muscles are the ones you use to stop the flow of urine when you're peeing or to clench your vagina. If your pelvic floor muscles are stronger it can be easier to prevent involuntary leaks when the pressure on your abdomen increases. There are several ways to train your pelvic floor muscles, but mainly this involves contracting the muscles in your genitals at intervals, the same way you train any other muscles at the gym. Many women get help from their GP or a physiotherapist. There are special exercise programs you can follow, including dedicated apps specially designed for pelvic floor training. You can also try vaginal balls or similar tools. The point of vaginal balls is to use your pelvic floor muscles to keep the balls in place for as long as you can manage. Regardless of how you exercise you will hopefully notice that you get stronger and have fewer leakages over time.

Pelvic floor exercises may also have some effect for women who suffer primarily from urge incontinence, but a process called bladder training is even more important. For those with urge incontinence, the bladder muscle contracts at the wrong time, without you having any control over it. That's why people often urinate such large amounts when they have urge incontinence. Bladder training is about teaching yourself to pee less frequently. The point is to urinate according to a time schedule and not according to need. You can start by saying that you're allowed to pee, say, once every hour. If a sudden urge arises between these permitted urination times, you must hold it in instead of running off to the bathroom. After a while you gradually increase the interval between each time you're allowed to relieve yourself, to two hours, three hours, four hours, and so on. Over time this will often help with urge incontinence.

In some cases medical treatment or surgery may be used to treat incontinence. For some women simple outpatient procedures make a world of difference, but for others exercise alone will do the trick. What helps you best will be a matter of what you yourself want and how serious your leakage problem is.

HEMORRHOIDS AND ANAL SKIN TAGS

Your anus, which must be able to expand a great deal, has a wrinkled appearance because of the sphincters that clamp the hole together. Its extra diameter is hidden by a structure akin to a pleated skirt. Normally, the pleats are evenly distributed around the hole to form a relatively flat surface. Not surprisingly, it can strike horror in your heart when you suddenly discover something new and alien hanging out of your butt. You feel as if the new protrusion is screaming out for attention, drawing the gaze toward a hole that a lot of people try to forget about entirely. Most likely, it's an anal skin tag or a hemorrhoid, both of which are harmless conditions.

Hemorrhoids are a common problem for both women and men. In fact, around a third of all adults have hemorrhoids although they're still not a common dinnertime topic, surprisingly enough.[85] It's possible to have them both inside the rectum and outside, around the anus; but let's stick to the external ones. A hemorrhoid is a hemorrhoid, regardless.

A hemorrhoid is a varicose vein in the anus and in appearance it is a balloon-like purplish-blue protrusion. You'll almost always be able to push it back into place again, unlike an anal skin tag, but then it'll pop out again the next time you defecate or do a particularly effortful squat. It can often be very itchy and maybe even painful. Sometimes the only problem may be that you'll find fresh blood on the toilet paper when you wipe. This is caused by the simple fact that a hemorrhoid is a blood vessel that's gone astray. Usually the blood vessels around the rectal opening are supported by connective tissue and mucous membranes, so we don't see them at all. With age, these supportive structures become flabbier and so increased pressure in the pelvis—for example straining on the toilet, heavy lifting, pregnancy, and childbirth—can cause a small section of a blood vessel to be pushed out of place, like a kink in a garden hose. Blood can then accumulate in this kink, forming a little balloon. The balloon is what we call a hemorrhoid.

Hemorrhoids around the butt are not dangerous, but they can be a real nuisance. Blood vessels don't like being messed with in this way, so small inflammations can easily arise around the hemorrhoid. Then you may find you get a bit of mucous, or that it's painful or itchy, so that the mere act of sitting—let alone emptying your bowels—becomes a tiresome business. Some people also find they bleed, either a little or a lot.

Fortunately, help is available. The most important thing to do, banal as it may sound, is ensure that you have good bathroom habits. Drink enough water to keep your feces soft and go to the bathroom only when you feel an urgent need, to avoid straining. We also recommend leaving your newspaper on the kitchen table. If you sit on the toilet for a long time the pressure around the hemorrhoid increases, which can worsen the problem. Good bathroom habits are often all it takes for hemorrhoids to slip back into place of their own accord. It's also sensible to push the hemorrhoid back into place with your finger when it pops out, so that it has a chance to find its way back to the right spot. It may feel a bit odd poking your finger in your butt like that, but if it's any consolation, doctors do this to total strangers every day of the week.

You can also buy various hemorrhoid creams at the pharmacy and these tend to work well. If that doesn't do the trick there are plenty of good treatment options your doctor can help you with, including surgery. And as you may have grasped by now, your doctor is used to doing this!

If the thing sticking out of your butt isn't a hemorrhoid, it's probably an anal skin tag. This is simply a slightly larger fold of skin in the anus, which is usually produced by the collapse of a hemorrhoid. When a hemorrhoid forces its way out, this can cause some of the folds of skin in the anal ring to come away from their proper place. Later, when the hemorrhoid retreats, they will combine to form a slightly larger fold that may protrude from the surface. An anal skin tag or two rarely causes major problems, although you may have temporary itching and secretions if the skin fold becomes irritated by chafing, say from wearing G-strings or having frequent bowel movements. Some people may find it more difficult to keep their butt clean.

However, some people feel that anal skin tags are aesthetically unsightly. It *is* possible to remove these tags surgically, but you should always give it a lot of thought before opting for a surgical procedure because there's a risk of complications. It's also worth being aware that removal hurts. You'll get a surgical scar in the middle of your butt, and, unfortunately, excrement isn't going to hold off because you've just had surgery. Our advice is to relax and leave the anal skin tags in peace unless they cause lots of problems.

CERVICAL CANCER AND HOW TO AVOID IT

The neck of the womb, or the cervix uteri, is the gateway between the uterus and the vagina. You can feel your cervix in the uppermost part of your vagina, like a stopper with the firmness of the tip of a nose, and with a tiny hole in the middle. This is the narrow channel the sperm cells travel through to reach the uterus. Your period comes out of here, and when you give birth your cervix can expand enough to let a whole baby pass through. It is also here that you can get cervical cancer.

Cervical cancer is unique among cancers. As early as the 1800s it was discovered that this type of cancer behaved differently from others. It was much more common among prostitutes than married women, and nuns were more or less spared the disease. Could it be a divine punishment for promiscuous women?

Nowadays we know that God and punishment have little to do with the matter. A viral disease that is transmitted through sex causes cervical cancer. We've mentioned this virus earlier in connection with sexually transmitted infections: human papillomavirus (HPV).

HPV is a large family of viruses, several of which give humans warts. Most of them are harmless—ordinary skin warts are caused by one type, for example. Some HPV types thrive best in the genitals. They are transmitted through sexual contact and most of us who are sexually active will be infected with one type or another over the course of our lives. More than 80 percent have had the virus before they turn fifty. HPV is therefore considered to be the most common venereal disease[86] and almost half of all people between twenty and twenty-four are walking around with an infection at any given time.[87]

As a rule, there's no cause for concern. Unlike with a herpes infection, your body will most often get rid of the virus on its own, the way it does with a cold. We know this because women who are checked for HPV over time often switch virus type. This indicates that the infections are short-lived and that women are reinfected with new virus types when they change partners.

However, certain types of HPV can give some people a prolonged infection of the cervix. These types are called high-risk viruses, and the most common ones are HPV 16 and 18. Over time, an infection like this can develop into cancer. Number 16 alone accounts for more than half of the cases of cervical cancer and may also cause mouth and throat cancer as well as vaginal, vulval, and anal cancer. However, the development of cancer requires more than an infection. It's common to be infected with HPV 16, but very few people get cancer. This means that other factors are decisive for the development of cancer—for example, special vulnerabilities in the person infected or other environmental factors such as smoking. What these other factors are, we do not yet know.

Put slightly differently, almost all the people who get cervical cancer have an infection caused by the HPV virus, but very few of those with an infection get cancer.

A LONG ROAD FROM SEX TO CANCER

Fortunately, cancer doesn't develop overnight. First the virus will cause you to have cell changes, or *dysplasia*, to use the technical term, in the cervix. This involves cells with small defects and abnormalities that prevent them from behaving in a typical way. In the beginning these abnormal cells are only slightly different, but if the immune defenses leave them in peace they can start to stand out from the crowd. Over time the cells can become more and more altered, until they are completely unrecognizable and start to grow in places they shouldn't. Only then do they become cancer cells.

In most cases it takes at least ten to fifteen years between the first innocent cell changes and full-blown cervical cancer. In the meantime, it is assumed that there are various stages of cell changes. During each of these stages, cells may change their minds or be destroyed by the immune system.

These kinds of cell changes, which *may* be precancerous stages, are the ones it's preferable to discover as early as possible. Through regular gynecological screening and cell tests every three years, changes can be identified and removed before they pose any threat. To defend effectively against cervical cancer, the screenings are a must.

Cell changes and cervical cancer rarely involve symptoms or signs that you are sick until late in the course of the disease. That's why examination of the cervix is so important. Symptoms of cervical cancer can include bleeding abnormalities, such as bleeding between periods or in connection with sex. Some women experience pain in their genitals or in their lower abdomen either during sex or in their day-to-day life. Others may find that their discharge starts to smell bad and contains traces of blood.

In other words, the signs that can accompany cervical cancer are very nonspecific: They are present in a lot of common and less harmful conditions of the genitals. If you have any of these symptoms, you should see your gynecologist for a checkup, but you shouldn't be worried about cancer. What you're experiencing is most likely a treatable venereal disease, a side effect of contraception, or a condition involving pain during sex—but it is important to check.

GET CHECKED

The Pap test is a simple solution for preventing cervical cancer. Women who have regular Pap tests reduce the risk of developing cervical cancer by 70 percent over their lifetime. That's what we call cheap life insurance. The American Cancer Society recommends that women should begin cervical cancer screening at age twenty-one. There is no need to get checked earlier, because cancer usually takes years to develop and the incidence of cancer in this age group is extremely low. Women aged twenty-one to twenty-nine should have a Pap test every three years.

Beginning at age thirty, the preferred screening method is a Pap test combined with an HPV test every five years. This is called co-testing and should continue until age sixty-five. Another reasonable option for women thirty to sixty-five is to get tested every three years with just the Pap test.

Getting a Pap test itself involves making an appointment with your gynecologist. You shouldn't take a Pap test during your period, and you should preferably not have had vaginal sex in the two days before the test. The gynecological examination takes just a few minutes. The doctor dilates your vagina with a kind of funnel called a speculum, looks at your cervix, and takes a sample with a little brush. The brush is rubbed gently against the cervix, loosening some cells that can then be examined under a microscope at the laboratory. If the cervical cells show abnormalities, you'll hear from your doctor within a week or two. If everything is normal you generally won't hear anything.

CELL CHANGES DON'T MEAN YOU HAVE CANCER

After a Pap test, you may get a confusing phone call from your doctor. You have abnormal cells—but what the heck does that mean?

A repeated theme among women we meet is that they are frustrated and anxious about inadequate information from their doctor when it comes to the process surrounding cell changes in the cervix. Most young women who are found to have abnormal cells feel perfectly healthy and have never thought they might get cancer. The news can come as much more of a shock than health professionals realize.

Many women become afraid that they already have cancer and will die if they're told cell changes have been found. What we would emphasize to such women is that it is very common for young and sexually active women to have slight cell changes in their cervix. Any HPV infection, even the low-risk viruses, may cause changes. This is why women under twenty-one aren't checked and why it's not recommended to do Pap tests more often than every three years—incredible numbers would become unnecessarily anxious and might end up being overtreated without improving our ability to pick up new cases of cancer.

In the vast majority of cases, cell changes in the cervix will disappear on their own without any kind of treatment. Like other viruses, HPV tends to pass. The body's own immune defenses are actually fantastic at tidying things up themselves! Your doctor knows this, which explains why she might not seem especially worried when all you can think about is CANCER.

Just to reassure you a bit more: 20 percent of American women aged twenty-five to fifty-four report a history of at least one previous abnormal Pap test. Just under 13,000 women are diagnosed with cervical cancer annually in the United States—and the five-year survival rate is 69 percent.

Let's take a look at what happened since you took your Pap test. The cells that were brushed off your cervix were sent to a laboratory. There, a doctor stained the cells and placed them under a microscope. The doctor looks for cells that appear abnormal. Depending on how unusual the cells look and how many of them there are, the cell changes are classified from mild to moderate and severe. Even serious cell changes can disappear of their own accord, but it's still important for all cell changes to be followed up.

As well as looking at the cells, the laboratory may examine the sample by applying an HPV test. Where on the scale the cell changes lie and the result of the HPV test are decisive elements when it comes to what happens next.

THE CELL SAMPLE SHOWS UNCERTAIN OR LOW-GRADE CELL CHANGES

You'll need to go back to your doctor for a control test six months later. By then the abnormal cells have most often repaired themselves after the virus attack or have been killed by your immune defenses. If the cell changes have retreated and the HPV test is negative, you're just as healthy as before and it will be three years until you'll need to take another Pap test. If you still have cell changes when you take the control test and if the HPV test came out positive, you'll need a more in-depth examination.

THE CELL SAMPLE SHOWS HIGH-GRADE OR SERIOUS CELL CHANGES

Your gynecologist will do two things. First, she will take a look at your cervix with a special magnifying instrument while you're set up in the stirrups on the exam table. This examination is called a *colposcopy* and is done to look for changes in the mucous membrane. After that, the gynecologist will take a tissue sample (*biopsy*) from your cervix, which will be sent to an expert—a pathologist—for examination under a microscope. During the cell test only a few cells are brushed off the surface of the mucous membrane, but in a biopsy a small piece of the cervix is removed to investigate whether there are abnormal cells deep in the mucous membrane. The whole architecture of the mucous membrane is examined.

Normally, you'll be given local anesthetic in your cervix, but it may hurt during and after the biopsy. Your gynecologist will likely advise you to take some ibuprofen ahead of the procedure. It is also normal to bleed a bit after the biopsy, so most women need to use a pad (not a tampon!) for the rest of the day.

When the pathologist examines the biopsy under the micro-scope, the changes will again be classified according to stages, from light to moderate to severe changes. None of these are cancer. Only when the abnormal cells have made their way through the mucous membrane is it a question of cervical cancer.

If the colposcopy and the biopsy are totally normal or show only slight changes, you can relax. However, you'll have to visit your gynecologist for a new Pap test and HPV test within six to twelve months to check that everything is fine. In nine out of ten cases, the changes will have vanished or remained stable without any kind of deterioration.[88]*

If any of the examinations confirm that there are moderate to severe precancerous stages, you will, as a rule, have a minor out-patient procedure called a cone biopsy. The outer part of the cervix is removed, normally with an electrical loop or sling. Previously doctors would perform a cone biopsy using a knife and then the part that was removed looked like an upside-down ice cream cone, which explains the name of the procedure. Now the portion of tissue that is removed looks more like a flat doughnut.

The cone biopsy is usually performed under local anesthetic, although some people may be given light general anesthesia. It's a simple procedure, but it isn't done unless necessary. This is because women who have had a cone biopsy have been observed to have a slightly higher risk of premature birth or miscarriage in subsequent pregnancies.

The vast majority of women who have had a cone biopsy, around 90 percent, will be totally cured. To be 100 percent certain, they are checked to make sure everything is fine, taking a new Pap test and HPV test six, twelve, and eighteen months after the procedure.

If the cell changes have gone away on their own or have been removed through a cone biopsy, there's no need to worry about cervical cancer. You have a clean slate.

---

* 60 percent of slight changes disappear spontaneously, while 30 percent remain stable. Only 10 percent will develop further into severe changes and 1 percent will develop into cancer over the person's lifetime.

Nonetheless it's important to remember that you can be infected with HPV again, so it may be a good idea to have the HPV vaccine (see "A Vaccine Against Cancer"). You must also continue to have screenings involving Pap tests every three years until you are sixty-five. But overall you should focus on not getting worked up about the prospect of cancer if one of your screenings shows abnormal cells.

A VACCINE AGAINST CANCER

We've discussed how you should have cell changes caused by the human papillomavirus treated, but imagine if you could prevent infection with the carcinogenic virus in the first place! A few years ago it would have seemed like science fiction, but today there actually is a vaccine that can protect against cancer. It's a medical miracle.

As we explained earlier, there are more than one hundred different types of HPV, but only a few of them cause cancer. There are three vaccines available the United States[89] designed to protect against the most dangerous types of HPV, numbers 16 and 18: Gardasil, Gardasil 9, and Cervarix.

Gardasil also protects against types 6 and 11, which cause 90 percent of cases of genital warts. Some studies show that Cervarix offers partial protection against genital warts too. It's important to grasp that there's no connection whatsoever between genital warts and cervical cancer, but I think we can all agree it's great to avoid them. Gardasil 9 protects against another five types of HPV (types 31, 33, 45, 52, and 58) that can lead to cancer of the cervix, anus, vulva, vagina, and mouth.

HPV vaccines are given in a series of shots over six months. If you're fifteen to twenty-six, the HPV vaccine is administered in three separate shots. The second shot is given two months after the first, and the third shot is given four months after the second shot.

For young people aged nine to fourteen, only two shots are needed. The second shot is given six months after the first.

Vaccination against these viruses gives young women almost 100 percent protection against infection and therefore against the cell changes and cervical cancer caused by these virus types. As a result of this, the Gardasil and Cervarix vaccines can prevent over 70 percent of cervical cancers, and Gardasil 9 can prevent 90 percent!

Since 2009, the HPV vaccine has formed part of Norway's child vaccination program. In other words, all girls are offered free vaccination when they are eleven to twelve years old. In the United States, the Center for Disease Control recommends the HPV vaccine for all young women aged eleven to twenty-six, and young men up to twenty-one, but it's up to parents to decide whether or not to have their children vaccinated. The HPV vaccine is not on the required list of vaccinations for US public school children.

A vaccine is not a medicine but a preventative shot that inhibits a virus from settling in your body and making you sick in the event of future infection. The vaccine stimulates the immune defenses to recognize the virus and prepare a battle plan for the quickest and most efficient means of crushing the virus if it should make an appearance. If you already have an ongoing HPV infection involving type 16 or 18, the vaccine will not eliminate the virus from your body. This is why the vaccine is given to young girls. It's imperative to protect them *before* they start having sex and potentially become infected with viruses.

The vaccine is approved for girls and boys aged seven to twenty-six, and has proven effective up to the age of forty-five. There are two reasons for this. First, very few of us are infected with *both* HPV 16 and 18. If you haven't yet been infected by these types, the vaccine will have a protective effect. Second, most HPV infections pass of their own accord. Unfortunately, it has been observed that natural immunization against HPV is poor. This means that even if you've had an earlier HPV infection, you're not necessarily protected against subsequent reinfection by a different sexual partner. An HPV vaccine can help protect you against this kind of reinfection.

The CDC recommends the HPV vaccines for both girls and boys, although much of the emphasis is placed on vaccinating girls, since they are the ones who risk developing cervical cancer. It should be just as effective for men—on genital warts and the more rare HPV-associated cancer of the penis, anus, and throat/ mouth—as it is for women. Some have observed a recent increase in throat and mouth cancer among men. There is speculation that this is because oral sex has become more common, causing men to be infected with oral HPV. A vaccine can prevent infection and the development of cancer here, too. Homosexual teenagers in particular should consider the vaccine since they are not indirectly protected by the more widespread vaccination of girls, often known as herd immunity.

For every sexual partner you have, the risk of HPV infection is around 10 percent. Even if you've already been infected with one or more types, it's very possible that you've never been infected by HPV 16 or 18. If you take the vaccine, you'll be protected against future infection by new sexual partners. As we mentioned, studies have shown that the vaccine is effective for women up to the age of forty-five. Put simply, this means that the number of sexual partners you've had is significant. The fewer previous partners, the greater the likelihood the vaccine will be effective for you. The number of sexual partners you end up having in the future will also play a role. The more of them there are, the greater the potential risk of infection and the greater the benefit of the vaccine. In addition, women who have been treated for abnormal cells have a lower risk of recurrence if they have received the HPV vaccine.

THE VACCINE IS SAFE AND EFFECTIVE

Today in Norway one in four twelve-year-old girls opt not to receive the free HPV vaccine.[90] We don't know why people choose to drop the vaccine but fear of side effects appears to be widespread. There are also some parents who think their twelve-year-old daughter won't have sex for many years and so the HPV vaccine is unnecessary. In Denmark there's been a great deal of media attention around possible side effects, and this has led to a drastic reduction in the proportion of vaccinated girls.[91]

In the United States, skepticism and even controversy persists regarding the HPV vaccine. A 2016 survey polled 1,501 parents of eleven- to seventeen-year-old children about their feelings concerning the HPV vaccine and found that only 40 percent believed the HPV vaccine prevented cervical cancer. Nearly 25 percent of the surveyed parents inaccurately believed the vaccine might cause long-term health problems, and one-third thought drug companies were pushing it to increase profits. One-third felt they lacked enough information to decide whether to vaccinate their children, and just 21 percent of parents believed laws requiring the HPV vaccine were a good idea, though that figure jumped to 57 percent if parents could opt out of the requirement.[92]

In Norway nearly 500,000 doses of the vaccine have been given to 160,000 girls. Within this total, 645 cases of possible side effects have been reported, 92 percent of which were described as nonserious. It was a matter of passing problems such as swelling and tenderness around the site of vaccination, fever, nausea, and diarrhea.

Of the few serious side effects reported since 2009, fifty-two in total, there are ten cases of chronic fatigue syndrome and five cases of postural orthostatic tachycardia syndrome (POTS). POTS is a condition that causes an elevated pulse rate when you stand up, as well as unstable blood pressure, fatigue, and dizziness. The Norwegian Medicines Agency reports that the number of cases is no higher than one would expect in this age group with or without the vaccine,[93] and a recent Norwegian study of 175,000 girls showed no increased rate of chronic fatigue syndrome among vaccinated girls.[94] In other words, the vaccine is not believed to have caused these problems.

Nonetheless, these kinds of reports about possible serious side effects are always taken extremely seriously. After many cases of conditions such as POTS were reported in Denmark after vaccination, the European Medical Agency decided to carry out a safety review. The result of the investigation came in November 2015. The conclusion was that no data point toward any causal link between the HPV vaccine and either POTS or another syndrome called CRPS (complex regional pain syndrome).[95] These are rare conditions, and their occurrence is no higher among vaccinated girls than in the rest of the population. Again, no link was found between the vaccine and chronic fatigue syndrome. More recently, a large cohort study of 3.1 million adult Danish and Swedish women found no association between the HPV vaccine and forty-four serious, chronic illnesses, including autoimmune diseases and neurological disease. The only association found was with celiac disease, although the researchers only found this in the Danish women.[96]

So far more than 180 million women worldwide have been vaccinated against HPV, and no serious safety problems have been proven to be connected with the vaccines. Although there will always be a possibility of side effects when using medication and vaccines, these tend to be mild, temporary problems. The same cannot be said of cervical cancer.

MISCARRIAGE–FROM FACEBOOK TO REALITY

In summer 2015 Mark Zuckerberg, the founder of Facebook, posted a slightly unusual update to his 33 million Facebook friends.[97] He and his wife, who is a pediatrician, announced that they were overjoyed to be expecting their first child, a girl, and were ready to make the world a better place for her sake. *Yawn*, you may think, automatically clicking Like. These sorts of personal announcements are commonplace on Facebook, a site that has become synonymous with humble bragging and image crafting.

But Zuckerberg didn't stop there. He chose to tell his followers about the rocky road to pregnancy—a story about everything we don't normally mention. The couple suffered three miscarriages over several years of trying to become parents. Four pregnancies resulted in one child (and 1.6 million Likes).

A miscarriage is a pregnancy that is involuntarily terminated before week twenty, when the fertilized egg stops developing or the fetus dies in the womb. You'll most often notice that you're miscarrying because you experience pain and vaginal bleeding. That said, there's nothing particularly unusual about bleeding during pregnancy. Around one in four pregnant women bleed in their first trimester, although miscarriage only occurs in one out of ten cases of bleeding.[98] Even so, you should always contact your obstetrician for a checkup if you bleed during pregnancy.

Miscarriage is one of the most common complications in early pregnancy. It happens in around one out of five *clinical* pregnancies, i.e., pregnancies that women themselves are aware of.[99] There are also miscarriages that happen before a pregnancy test can detect that you're pregnant. These types of pregnancies are generally called chemical pregnancies. Taking chemical pregnancies into account, it is assumed that only half of all fertilized eggs will result in viable pregnancies.[100] In other words, miscarriage is as common as a successful pregnancy.

Pregnancy tests today are so sensitive that they can detect you're pregnant incredibly early, but it's not necessarily wise to use this option if you're hoping for a positive result—because most miscarriages happen in the first few weeks after fertilization, before your next period is due. Since it's so common for these early pregnancies to end in miscarriage, you can save yourself a great deal of disappointment by waiting to take the test until after the point you were expecting to have your period. If you wait two extra weeks, until week six of the pregnancy, the risk of miscarriage has fallen to 10 to 15 percent. A positive result at that point therefore implies that you'll probably be a mother in eight months' time. After eight weeks, the risk is down to just three percent. Once the three-month mark is past, the risk stabilizes at a low level of around 0.6 percent.[101] With every passing week, the chances that everything will be fine become higher and higher.

Fear of miscarriage is the reason why women often choose to wait until the first trimester is out of the way before telling people about their pregnancy. The idea behind this secrecy is primarily to spare the pregnant woman in case anything goes wrong. It's bad enough to lose a longed-for baby without also having to tell friends and family to call off the happy news. It's debatable whether three months is a sensible limit. You could just as well set the limit one month earlier, around week eight, if you have to have a limit at all.

Unfortunately, the result of this secrecy is that many couples feel there's something shameful about miscarriage. It's not unusual to hear people commenting after a miscarriage: "Well, it was a bit odd to tell people so soon," as if you could kill the fetus in your womb just by talking about it. It's quite absurd. Zuckerberg described miscarriage as a lonely experience: "Most people don't discuss miscarriages because you worry your problems will distance you or reflect upon you—as if you're defective or did something to cause this. So you struggle on your own."

Zuckerberg isn't alone in these feelings. In a study published in *Obstetrics & Gynecology*, nearly half of those who had been through a miscarriage reported feeling that they were somehow to blame, or having a sense that they had done something wrong. They felt alone and ashamed.[102] It makes for sad reading, not least because self-blame is caused by a relatively widespread misunderstanding of the causes of miscarriage. In the same study, it emerged that almost a quarter thought that lifestyle choices, such as smoking, alcohol, and drugs, were the most *common* cause of miscarriage. Many people also thought that heavy lifting and stress could lead to miscarriage. On mother and baby forums online, coffee drinking and bubble baths are named as other possible causes.

In reality, miscarriage is rarely a result of missteps by the mother (or father). The most common cause of miscarriage is serious chromosomal abnormality in the fetus, i.e., an error in the genetic code that has already been determined at conception. Forget the boozing, unhealthy eating, or social smoking you indulged in before you knew you were pregnant.

The merging of the mother's and father's genetic material into a joint recipe for a unique person, which must be followed to the letter, is inconceivably complicated. It's not surprising that errors happen frequently for no good reason. Miscarriage is the body's control mechanism and its way of ensuring that we have healthy children who can live good lives. It can be horribly painful to suffer a miscarriage like this, but it's actually your body doing right by you.

Only when you've had two or three in a row should you consider investigating whether there's something in the mother (or father) that is causing the miscarriages. Before that, it's seen as a very normal occurrence. Where women experience repeated miscarriages, the cause can be anything from anatomical aberrations and hormonal disorders to autoimmune diseases and hereditary blood conditions. These are conditions nobody can be blamed for but that hopefully can be treated.

Simple bad luck is the most frequent cause of miscarriage, but we do know that a few things increase the risk. The most important factor is the mother's age. A Danish study found that 25 percent of all pregnancies in thirty-five- to thirty-nine-year-olds ended in miscarriage, compared with 12 percent among twenty-five- to twenty-nine-year-olds.[103] By the age of forty only half of pregnancies ended in birth, mostly, but not solely, because the quality of the eggs starts to become so poor that errors in chromosomes and genes that make the fetus nonviable are more frequent.

We all know there's no place for smoking in a pregnancy. You should stop smoking as soon as you know you're pregnant. But what about the time before you find out? What about that time you smoked at a party when you still didn't know? The biggest review of research that has been undertaken found a clear link between smoking and miscarriage.[104] If a hundred nonsmokers and a hundred smokers became pregnant, twenty of those in the first group would miscarry versus around twenty-six among the smokers.* It is estimated that around one in ten miscarriages are caused by smoking,[105] but it seems as if you have to smoke a great deal—more than ten cigarettes a day—in order to appreciably increase the risk.[106]

---

* The relative risk of miscarriage during pregnancy was 1.32 for smokers compared with nonsmokers. In this example we have assumed that the risk of miscarriage for nonsmokers is 20 percent. This may well be too high, but has been chosen to illustrate relative risk in an understandable way.

So a little bit of social smoking in the first few weeks shouldn't be grounds for deep guilt or anxiety.

The same is true of alcohol to a certain extent. Alcohol is extremely harmful for a fetus, but we don't know how much it takes to cause damage. It's not easy to check how much pregnant women can drink before the fetus suffers damage or death. It would be incredibly unethical to ask a group of pregnant women to drink during pregnancy to check how much alcohol was needed to cause miscarriage or fetal injury. Since we don't know where the limit lies, health care professionals recommend avoiding alcohol entirely. That way you'll be on the safe side.

However, not everybody agrees that total abstinence from alcohol is the only right way, and this can be confusing when you're pregnant. Nina discovered this herself when she was pregnant and many doctors told her a glass of red wine now and then was perfectly fine. The world-famous economist Emily Oster got sick of these mixed messages and decided to investigate the research behind the advice more closely. In her book *Expecting Better—Why the Conventional Pregnancy Wisdom Is Wrong and What You Really Need to Know* (2013), Oster claims there is little to support official advice about the *absolute* avoidance of alcohol in pregnancy.[107] Her analysis indicates that it's safe to drink one to two units of alcohol a week, i.e., a small glass of wine or one glass of beer on two different days of the week won't have long-term effects on a child's behavior or intelligence. In her view, the official advice to totally abstain from alcohol is driven by the assumption that women won't be able to limit themselves: If you accept a glass of wine on your birthday, it'll quickly become a whole bottle. We agree with Oster that this underestimates women's self-discipline; most of us manage to stop drinking for the full nine months, after all.

But perhaps it isn't that one glass of red wine with dinner you're worrying about when your pregnancy test comes out positive. Many women get nervous when they find out they're pregnant because of a slightly too drunk party in the weeks before, where a lot more than one or two glasses of alcohol were consumed. A

Danish population-based study from 2012 found that the risk of miscarriage doubled if women had four or more drinks a week in the first three months of their pregnancy.[108] In theory, therefore, a real bender in the weeks before you discover your pregnancy can lead to miscarriage, but this by no means implies that it will necessarily happen. And if it does, it's impossible to put a finger on whether your boozing session was the specific cause. The miscarriage might have happened anyway. Just think how incredibly common it is!

Now on to the rumors that abound on the Internet: heavy lifting, stress, and normal amounts of coffee drinking do not lead to miscarriage. It seems that you'd have to drink ten cups of coffee a day before it *might* constitute a risk.[109] Cross-country skiing champion Marit Bjørgen trained for six hours a day during pregnancy and delivered her baby just fine. Nor does it seem that vitamin supplements can protect against miscarriage,[110] although you should start taking folic acid, which is a B vitamin, from the moment you find out you're pregnant—and preferably from the time you start trying to get pregnant. It can prevent damage to your child's nervous system.

Sharing our lives on social media is widespread these days. A lot of people think it's too intimate and compromising to talk about pregnancy-related experiences in public spaces, but as we saw in Mark Zuckerberg's post about his family, there are indeed important messages to share. Openness about miscarriage helps to make clear just how common it actually is, as well as the fact that it's an event that affects all kinds of people. There's nothing shameful about a miscarriage and it's usually nobody's fault. The vast majority of people who have miscarriages go on to have totally healthy children later.

The three-month rule we mentioned earlier was intended to protect women against the pain of telling others about the miscarriage, but perhaps this rule actually does more harm than good. It can perpetuate misunderstandings and stigma instead of normalizing and creating acceptance. The result is that many women are left feeling isolated, with an unjustified sense of shame and guilt, at a time when they're most in need of support and consideration from the people around them. Let's start talking to each other!

THE TICKING CLOCK—HOW LONG CAN YOU PUT OFF HAVING CHILDREN?

When you're approaching thirty, it's weird how often strangers feel they have the right to get involved in your private life. "The clock's ticking! Isn't it about time you started thinking about having children?" It's irrelevant to them whether you're single, in a new relationship, or married to your job. They'd rather see you drop everything you're doing and force the first man you can lay your hands on to engage in immediate reproduction.

Think about having children, sure. A lot of women think and think without any children coming of it. Even if you want to have children—which is absolutely not a given—there are plenty of potential obstacles. The most obvious one is finding a person you can actually imagine having children with and who is also ready to have children with you. Oddly enough, a lot of men head for the hills the minute a sweet young woman in a bar starts talking about strollers and settling down with stars in her eyes after the second drink.

Unfortunately, we can't help you find the perfect dad, but what we can do is give you a little ammunition to use on those busybodies who won't stop talking about babies. Or a dose of reassurance if you're starting to feel stressed.

Let's start with a few facts. Around 75 percent of all couples who try to get pregnant manage it within six months. Before the year is over, somewhere between 85 and 90 percent will have gotten pregnant.[111] *Infertility* is defined as an absence of pregnancy after a year of regular unprotected sex. This term applies to around 10 to 15 percent of all couples, but that's not the end of it. Of the couples who have been labeled infertile, half will become pregnant quite naturally in the course of the second year of trying. They should, in fact, be called *subfertile*. They struggle to have children, but achieve it if they try for long enough. In all, up to 95 percent of all heterosexual people manage to have children through regular intercourse given plenty of time.

And then there's the matter of age. The average age for first births has steadily risen as women have entered and become more prominent in the workforce. In 2014, women in Oslo had their first child at age 30.8, on average.[112] In the United States between 2000 and 2014, the mean age of first-time mothers increased from 24.9 years to 26.3.[113] Women want to wait longer before having children than they used to both because they go to school for longer and want to build a career. At the same time, the medical community issues us with warnings, highlighting figures that show a dramatic drop in fertility as we age and urging us to think carefully before we put off trying to get pregnant. There are several good reasons for this—among others, the risk of complications in pregnancy and abnormalities in children increases as the mother becomes older—we'll come back to that (page 272). The question is whether we exaggerate the difficulties of having children once we hit our thirtieth birthday.

Several more recent studies have examined healthy women and their likelihood of getting pregnant. Although fewer women become spontaneously pregnant as they get older, the figures are less dramatic than you might imagine. One study followed 782 couples who were trying to have a child.[114] The women in the nineteen to twenty-six age group were clearly most fertile—92 percent got pregnant within a year—and after that the trend declined. But no major differences were found between the fertility of women in their late twenties and those at the beginning of their thirties. For women between the ages of twenty-seven and thirty-four, 86 percent got pregnant within a year. By comparison, 82 percent of those between thirty-five and thirty-nine got pregnant in the same period. Other studies have found similar figures. In a Danish study of 3,000 women, 72 percent of all the thirty-five- to forty-year-olds got pregnant in the course of the year, while 78 percent of those who tried to time intercourse in relation to ovulation became pregnant. The figure for thirty- to thirty-four-year-olds was 87 percent.[115]

What can we take away from this? If all young women tried to get pregnant when they left high school, one in ten would fail. Twenty years later, this figure rises to somewhere between two and three out of ten. However, the upside is that the majority of all women manage to get pregnant well into their thirties!

For most people who are struggling to get pregnant, age is not a direct cause. First, we should point out that the problem lies with the man in a third of cases, because the man's age also plays a role. The woman is the problem, or a part of the problem, in the rest of the cases. What's wrong then? The biggest source of infertility is disorders in the hormones that control ovulation. It's often due to polycystic ovary syndrome, where the hormone balance is not as it should be. The next most common cause is damage to the fallopian tubes. This may be caused by past sexually transmitted infections, such as chlamydia, where the bacteria have caused inflammation and scarring of the fallopian tubes. The problems may also be caused by endometriosis, which is the condition where uterine lining grows in the wrong place. Finally, fibroids—i.e., myomas in the uterus—can prevent pregnancy. These are the most common causes of problems with pregnancy, not age.

However, the problem with increasing age is a higher risk of miscarriage. As we mentioned earlier, the risk of miscarriage is twice as high for women over thirty-five.[116] Naturally, this means that those over this age who are expecting children experience miscarriage more often than the women who get pregnant prior to age thirty-five.

Age has a clearly negative effect on your chances of getting pregnant, and the risk of miscarriage, pregnancy complications, and chromosomal errors such as Down syndrome increases. Still, the majority of women will not have any problem having healthy children "the old-fashioned way" well into their thirties. The likelihood that you're one of the women who will struggle is, of course, impossible to determine based on statistics, but it may be that you would have struggled to have children even if you'd tried at twenty-eight. If you suspect that you have endometriosis or polycystic ovary syndrome, or if you've had chlamydia several times, you may not want to postpone trying to get pregnant for too long. It might take some extra help and time to succeed.

GENITAL MUTILATION

Every year many millions of girls are mutilated for life. Their genitals are cut, sewn up, or pricked with needles. Genital mutilation is a cultural practice that exists in several corners of the world, but that is fortunately becoming less and less common. Today it occurs most frequently in parts of Africa, the Middle East, and certain Asian countries, but there was a time when people also practiced genital mutilation in the West. From the mid-1800s, many gynecologists in the United States and England cut away women's clitorises to prevent them from masturbating, because masturbation could, it was believed, lead to hysteria, epilepsy, and low IQ.[117] Cutting women's genitals has always been and continues to be a brutal effort to control female sexuality.

In Norway and the United States, a lot of effort has gone into preventing girls from an immigrant background from being mutilated and it seems that the work has been paying off. But for many women the damage is already done and that's why we've included this section. We also think it serves as a reminder of how female genitals are still considered a threat in large parts of the world.

The World Health Organization divides genital mutilation into four categories. The first involves removing the whole or parts of the clitoral nub, or glans. The clitoral hood is also often removed. One explanation that has often been given is the perception that the clitoris can grow into a kind of penis if it is not removed, but there's no getting away from the fact that by removing or damaging the clitoris, you're removing the principal source of women's sexual pleasure. It is an attempt to control our sexuality. Even so some women retain part of their sensation and capacity to have orgasms, because the clitoral complex mainly lies beneath the surface of the skin.* Other women find that the scar tissue produced in the clitoris creates constant pain.

The second form of genital mutilation involves cutting away the inner labia, often combined with various forms of damage to the clitoris. The inner labia grow when we reach puberty, in tandem with the sexual awakening of our teenage years. Perhaps people saw a connection between growth in the genitals and interest in sex. By removing the labia, they maintain the illusion of childish innocence.

The third form of female genital mutilation is the one that often gets the most attention, because it's the most aggressive alteration of the genitals. In this case, the outer labia are simply sewn together so all that's left is a small hole above the entrance to the vagina. Sometimes the inner labia and the clitoris are cut away at the same time. Both urine and menstrual blood seep out of this artificial opening. One Norwegian Somali woman we met told us what a shock it was to pee in a public toilet in Norway for the first time—the Norwegian women peed like elephants, she said! She was used to spending up to twenty minutes emptying her bladder, so sparse was her urine flow. The same problem can arise during menstruation, when the blood can accumulate in the vagina. That makes it a hotbed of bacteria, exposing women to genital and urinary tract infections.

The constructed hole is often too small for sexual intercourse, and therefore serves as a kind of guarantee that the woman hasn't had vaginal intercourse before she gets married. Of course, problems arise when she's due to have sex for the first time and risks having to be opened up with scissors or a knife, or being split open with the man's penis. Some women have a big enough hole to have penetrative sex, but must be opened up before they can give birth. The scar tissue around the vagina is unable to expand enough to let a baby through. If they are not opened up, they risk suffering

---

*   In the book *Bonk: The Curious Coupling of Science and Sex*, Mary Roach talks about the meetings between the researcher Marie Bonaparte and Egyptian women who had suffered genital mutilation but still masturbated by stimulating the scarred clitoris.

uncontrolled tears, creating the potential for heavy bleeding and damage to the rectum.

The last form of genital mutilation is a miscellaneous group that includes all the damage to the genitals that is not included in the other three groups. This can, for example, include sticking hot needles into the clitoris—a kind of ritual killing of a woman's sexuality.

All forms of genital mutilation can cause long-term problems of the genitals. In addition, the procedure itself is linked to a major risk of infections and bleeding, not to mention psychological trauma. There are good reasons why genital mutilation is strictly forbidden in many parts of the world. In Norway and the United States, all forms of female genital mutilation that can lead to long-term damage of the genitals are punishable by law, even if the girl or woman wants it herself. Neither is it permissible to take one's child overseas to have it done there.

However, there is no prohibition on being genitally mutilated. If you have previously been mutilated and have problems, you can get help. Doctors can carry out reconstructive surgery to try to normalize the function of your genitals. They can't give you back the genitals you were born with, but they can minimize your daily problems.

AFTERWORD

What a journey! We hope you've learned a lot and had a few surprises, as we most certainly have. Female genitals are fantastic. We really hope you're proud to have them. We also hope we've lit a spark in you, making you more curious and interested in your own genitals. As with all knowledge, there's always more to be acquired. What's more, medicine is a profession in a constant process of development, so we encourage you to never stop learning.

Unfortunately for many, their genitals are a source of mystery and shame. There's a whole world of genital problems, and even though our sophisticated reproductive system is designed to put up with a lot, sometimes we face dilemmas and disease, although at least we don't have to worry about being kicked in the balls. Genital problems can feel especially intimate and shameful. Few people speak openly about these issues, the way they talk about throat infections or slipped disks, leaving many women to feel alone and anxious when things aren't the way they usually are. We hope this book has given you the knowledge you need to visit your doctor with your head held high and that perhaps it's given you more confidence to know when to worry and when to chill out.

We also hope you've abandoned some of the negative thoughts you may have had about your genitals or your sex life. We've met a lot of women who feel abnormal because they don't have orgasms solely through vaginal penetration, or because they think they have genital herpes or a vulva that looks nothing like the illustrations in an anatomy book. As you've seen here, these misconceptions are very common.

In our sexualized daily lives it can sometimes be easy to forget that our bodies are about more than appearance and performance, and that a naked body isn't always about sex. It's too easy to base your self-worth on what you do in bed or the way you look. What we perceive as our shortcomings often become consuming. Your sex life should be on your own terms. The important thing is to learn to enjoy yourself and your body, just the way you are, both alone and with your partners. Not everybody gets to do everything, and not everybody looks the same. When it comes down to it, a body is just a body, but it's valuable because it's the only one you'll ever have.

ACKNOWLEDGMENTS

We'd like to thank some specially selected people. Marius Johansen has done a fantastic job of quality-assuring the medical aspect of the text, as well as being a brilliant guy and a brilliant doctor. We hope this won't be our last collaboration. Other wonderful professionals have also contributed their specialist knowledge. Thank you to Kjartan Moe, Trond Diseth, Kari Ormstad, Sveinung W. Sørbye, Jorun Thørring, Anne Lise Helgesen, Anders Røyneberg, Eszter Vanki, Berit Austveg, and Reidun Førde for the conversations, read-throughs, and comments. We must thank the professors at University of Oslo Medical Faculty who, without knowing it, have given us the answers we were wondering about during lectures or in patient conversations between classes. We must stress that any mistakes in this book are our responsibility entirely.

We would like to thank our former and current colleagues at Medisinernes Seksualopplysning Oslo, Stiftelsen SUSS-telefon, Sex og samfunn, and Olafiaklinikken for creating good, stimulating learning environments. We are unbelievably grateful to our dear friends and colleagues who have read and discussed and called us out when we've gotten tangled up in incomprehensible explanations.

Thanks to all of you who read our blog and those of you who've offered suggestions for topics, asked sensible questions, and cheered us on. We wrote this book for you.

An especially big thank-you to our editor, Nazneen Khan-Østrem at Aschehoug. It makes us so happy to discuss everything from periods to punk rock with you, and it's given us such a sense of security knowing that you were watching our backs. Thank you to TegneHanne, Hanne Sigbjørnsen, who has drawn the best illustrations we could imagine. It's been a gift having such a funny nurse on our team. Thank you also to the team at Quercus who have been so enthusiastic about bringing this book to the US market and adapting it from its Scandi roots.

And now, at last, there's no getting away from our families.

From Nina: This book was conceived at around the same time that my son came into the world. It wouldn't have been possible without the most patient and considerate boyfriend I could wish for, Fredrik. You're a whole lot of man per square meter. Mads, you're my little ray of sunshine and I'm sure you'll be horribly embarrassed when you read Mommy's book someday. I'll try not to talk too much about lady parts at the dinner table. Mom, Dad, and Helch—you are the best family a person could wish for.

From Ellen: Thanks to Mom, Dad, and Helge, the world's best family, who have patiently listened to long and pretty intense monologues about hymens, vulval pains, herpes, and other such dross—sometimes in public and inappropriate places. Thanks also to Grandfather, who compared us to Karl Evang, women's sexual health pioneer in Norway. I love you all beyond measure. Most of all I want to thank Henning, for more reasons than I feel inclined to write down.

Happy reading!
Nina and Ellen
Oslo, Norway

NOTES

1. Vigsnæs, M. K., K. Spets and C. Quist. "Politiet slår alarm: Grenseløs sexkultur blant barn og unge," *VG*, 2016; [updated 09/15/2016]. Available at: http://pluss.vg .no/2016/08/20/2508/2508_23770417.
2. Bergo, I. G. and C. Quist. "Kunnskapsministeren om sexkulturen blant unge: Skolen må ta mer ansvar," *VG*, 2016. Available at: http://www.vg.no/nyheter/ innenriks/kunnskapsministeren-om-sexkulturen-blant-unge-skolen-maa-ta-mer -ansvar/a/23770735/.

GENITALS

1. Boston University School of Medicine. "Female Genital Anatomy," *Sexual Medicine*, 2002. Available at: http://www.bumc.bu.edu/sexualmedicine/ physicianinformation/female-genital-anatomy/.
2. Kilchevsky, A., Y. Vardi, L. Lowenstein, and I. Gruenwald. "Is the Female G-Spot Truly a Distinct Anatomic Entity?," *Journal of Sexual Medicine*, 2012; 9(3):719–26.
3. Buisson, O., P. Foldes, E. Jannini, and S. Mimoun. "Coitus as Revealed by Ultra-sound in One Volunteer Couple," *Journal of Sexual Medicine*, 2010; 7(8):2750–4.
4. Darling, C. A., J. K. Davidson Sr., and C. Conway-Welch. "Female Ejaculation: Per-ceived Origins, the Grafenberg Spot/Area, and Sexual Responsiveness," *Archives of Sexual Behavior*, 1990; 19(1):29–47.
5. O'Connell, H. E. and J. O. DeLancey. "Clitoral Anatomy in Nulliparous, Healthy, Premenopausal Volunteers Using Unenhanced Magnetic Resonance Imaging," *Journal of Urology*, 2005; 173(6):2060–3.
6. O'Connell, H. E., K. V. Sanjeevan, and J. M. Hutson, "Anatomy of the Clitoris," *Journal of Urology*, 2005; 174(4 Pt. 1):1189–95.
7. Pauls, R. N. "Anatomy of the Clitoris and the Female Sexual Response," *Clinical Anatomy*, 2015; 28(3):376–84.
8. Lloyd, J., N. S. Crouch, C. L. Minto, L. M. Liao, and S. M. Creighton. "Female Genital Appearance: 'Normality' Unfolds," *BJOG*, 2005; 112(5):643–6.
9. Di Marino, V. and H. Lepidi. *Anatomic Study of the Clitoris and the Bulbo-clitoral Organ* (Springer International Publishing, 2014), 91.
10. Maravilla, K. A., J. R. Heiman, P. A. Garland, Y. Cao, B. T. Carter, W. O. Peterson, et al. "Dynamic MR Imaging of the Sexual Arousal Response in Women," *Journal of Sex & Marital Therapy*, 2003; 29:71–6.
11. Karacan, I., A. Rosenbloom, and R. Williams. "The Clitoral Erection Cycle during Sleep," *Journal of Sleep Research*, 1970.
12. Fisher, C., H. D. Cohen, R. C. Schiavi, D. Davis, B. Furman, K. Ward, et al. "Pat-terns of Female Sexual Arousal during Sleep and Waking: Vaginal Thermo-Conductance Studies," *Archives of Sexual Behavior*, 1983; 12(2):97–122.

13. Nesheim, B. I. "Deflorasjon," *Store Medisinske Leksikon*, 2009. Available at: https://sml.snl.no/deflorasjon.
14. Smith, A. "The Prepubertal Hymen," *Australian Family Physician*, 2011; 40(11):873.
15. Berenson, A., A. Heger, and S. Andrews. "Appearance of the Hymen in Newborns," *Pediatrics*, 1991; 87(4):458–65.
16. Whitley, N. "The First Coital Experience of One Hundred Women," *Journal of Obstetric, Gynecologic, and Neonatal Nursing*, 1978; 7(4):41–5.
17. Hägstad, A. J. "Mödomen—mest myt!," *Läkartidningen*, 1990; 87(37):2857–8.
18. Zariat, I. "Rystende jomfrusjekk," *NRK Ytring*, 2016; [updated 08/28/2016]. Available at: https://www.nrk.no/ytring/rystende-jomfrusjekk-1.13106033.
19. Independent Forensic Expert Group. "Statement on Virginity Testing," *Journal of Forensic and Legal Medicine*, 2015; 33:121–4.
20. Olson, R. and C. Garcia-Moreno. "Virginity Testing: A Systematic Review," *Reproductive Health*, May 18, 2017. Available at: https://doi.org/10.1186/s12978-017-0319-0.
21. Adams, J. A., A. S. Botash, and N. Kellogg. "Differences in Hymenal Morphology Between Adolescent Girls with and Without a History of Consensual Sexual Intercourse," *Archives of Pediatrics & Adolescent Medicine*, 2004; 158(3):280–5.
22. Kellogg, N. D., S. W. Menard, and A. Santos. "Genital Anatomy in Pregnant Adolescents: 'Normal' Does Not Mean 'Nothing Happened,'" *Pediatrics*, 2004; 113:67–9.
23. McCann, J., S. Miyamoto, C. Boyle, and K. Rogers. "Healing of Hymenal Injuries in Prepubertal and Adolescent Girls: A Descriptive Study," *Pediatrics*, 2007; 119(5):1094–1106.
24. Berenson, A. B., M. R. Chacko, C. M. Wiemann, C. O. Mishaw, W. N. Friedrich, and J. J. Grady. "Use of Hymenal Measurements in the Diagnosis of Previous Penetration," *Pediatrics*, 2002; 109(2):228–35.
25. Myhre, A. K., G. Borgen, and K. Ormstad. "Seksuelle overgrep mot prepubertale barn," *Tidsskrift for Den norske legeforening*, 2006; 126(19):2511.
26. Hasselknippe, O. and O. Stokke. "Volvat slutter å selge jomfruhinner," *Aftenposten*, 2006; [updated 10/19/2011]. Available at: http://www.aftenposten.no/norge/Volvat-slutter-a-selge-jomfruhinner-423873b.html.
27. Førde, R. "Operativ rekonstruksjon av jomfruhinne," *Tidsskrift for Den norske legeforening*, 2002.
28. The Hymen Shop. The Artificial Hymen Kit. Available at: http://www.hymenshop.com/.
29. "Egyptians Want to Ban Fake Virginity Kit," *Telegraph* (2009). Available at: http://www.telegraph.co.uk/news/worldnews/africaandindianocean/egypt/6264741/Egyptians-want-to-ban-fake-virginity-kit.html.
30. Paul, R. and G. Cotsarelis. "The Biology of Hair Follicles," *New England Journal of Medicine*, 1999; 341(7):491–7.
31. Olsen, E. A. "Methods of Hair Removal," *Journal of the American Academy of Dermatology*, 1999; 40:1433–55; 56–7.
32. Paul and Cotsarelis. "The Biology of Hair Follicles."
33. Shenenberger, D. W. "Removal of Unwanted Hair," Waltham, MA: *UpToDate*, 2016. Available at: https://uptodate.com/contents/removal-of-unwanted-hair.
34. Goldstein, B. G. and A. O. Goldstein. "Pseudofolliculitis Barbae," Waltham, MA: *UpToDate*, 2016. Available at: https://www.uptodate.com/contents/pseudofolliculitis-barbae.

35. Howarth, C., J. Hayes, M. Simonis, and M. Temple-Smith. "Everything's Neatly Tucked Away: Young Women's Views on Desirable Vulval Anatomy," *Culture, Health & Sexuality*, 2016:1–16.

36. Murakami, H. *Kafka on the Shore* (London: Vintage, 2005).

37. Wallace, W. H. B. and T. W. Kelsey. "Human Ovarian Reserve from Conception to the Menopause," *PLOS ONE*, 2010; 5(1):e8722.

38. Ibid.

39. Tanbo, T. G. Email from MD Tom Gunnar Tanbo, former consultant at the Section for Reproductive Medicine, Gynecology department, OUS, Oslo University Hospital, 2016.

40. http://bit.ly/menopauseorg.

DISCHARGE, PERIODS, AND OTHER GORE

1. Sobel, J. D. "Patient Education: Vaginal Discharge in Adult Women (Beyond the Basics)," Waltham, MA: *UpToDate*, 2016. Available at: https://www.uptodate.com/contents/vaginal-discharge-in-adult-women-beyond-the-basics.

2. Dyall-Smith, D. "Trimethylaminuria," *DermNet New Zealand*, 2016. Available at: http://www.dermnetnz.org/topics/trimethylaminuria/.

3. http://bit.ly/cdctricho.

4. Emera, D., R. Romero, and G. Wagner. "The Evolution of Menstruation: A New Model for Genetic Assimilation," *BioEssays*, 2012; 34(1):26–35.

5. Frank, L. "Blodig uenighet," *Morgenbladet*, June 10, 2016.

6. McClintock, M. K. "Menstrual Synchrony and Suppression," *Nature*, 1971; 229(5282):244.

7. Turke, P. W. "Effects of Ovulatory Concealment and Synchrony on Protohominid Mating Systems and Parental Roles," *Ethology and Sociobiology*, 1984; 5(1):33–4.

8. Arden, M., L. Dye, and A. Walker. "Menstrual Synchrony: Awareness and Subjective Experiences," *Journal of Reproductive and Infant Psychology*, 1999; 17(3):255–65.

9. Trevathan, W. R., M. H. Burleson, and W. L. Gregory. "No Evidence for Menstrual Synchrony in Lesbian Couples," *Psychoneuroendocrinology*, 1993; 18(5):425–35.

10. Yang, Z. and J. C. Schank. "Women Do Not Synchronize Their Menstrual Cycles," *Human Nature*, 2006; 17(4):433–47.

11. Dillner, L. "Do Women's Periods Really Synchronise When They Live Together?," *Guardian*, 2016; [updated 09/15/2016]. Available at: https://www.theguardian.com/lifeandstyle/2016/aug/15/periods-housemates-menstruation-synchronise.

12. Wikipedia. "Sanitary Napkin," *Wikipedia*, 2016; [updated 09/21/2016]. Available at: https://en.wikipedia.org/wiki/Sanitary_napkin.

13. NEL—Norsk elektronisk legehåndbok. "Toksisk sjokksyndrom (TSS)," *NEL*, 2014; [updated 01/22/2014]. Available at: https://legehandboka.no/handboken/kliniske-kapitler/infeksjoner/tilstander-og-sykdommer/bakteriesykdommer/toksisk-sjokk-syndrome/.

14. Mitchell, M. A., S. Bisch, S. Arntfield, and S. M. Hosseini-Moghaddam. "A Confirmed Case of Toxic Shock Syndrome Associated with the Use of a Menstrual Cup," *Canadian Journal of Infectious Diseases & Medical Microbiology*, 2015; 26(4):218–20.

15. NEL—Norsk elektronisk legehåndbok. "Premenstruelt syndrom," *NEL*, 2015; [updated 09/06/2015]. Available at: https://legehandboka.no/handboken/kliniske-kapitler/gynekologi/tilstander-og-sykdommer/menstruasjonsproblemer/premenstruelt-syndrome.

16. https://www.acog.org/Patients/FAQs/Premenstrual-Syndrome-PMS.
17. NEL. "Premenstruelt syndrome."
18. Yonkers, K. A., P. M. S. O'Brien, and E. Eriksson. "Premenstrual Syndrome," *Lancet*, 2008; 371(9619):1200–10.
19. Grady-Weliky, T. A. "Premenstrual Dysphoric Disorder," *New England Journal of Medicine*, 2003; 348(5):433–8.
20. https://www.uptodate.com/contents/clinical-manifestations-and-diagnosis-of -premenstrual-syndrome-and-premenstrual-dysphoric-disorder?source=search _result&search=PMS&selectedTitle=2~150.
21. NEL. "Premenstruelt syndrome."
22. Wilcox, A. J., C. R. Weinberg, and D. D. Baird. "Timing of Sexual Intercourse in Relation to Ovulation—Effects on the Probability of Conception, Survival of the Pregnancy and Sex of the Baby," *New England Journal of Medicine*, 1995; 333(23):1517–21.

SEX

1. Træen, B., H. Stigum, and P. Magnus. *Rapport fra seksualvaneundersøkelsene i 1987, 1992, 1997, og 2002.* (Oslo: Statens institutt for folkehelse, 2003).
2. https://www.guttmacher.org/factsheet/american-teens-sexual-and-reproductive -health.
3. Træen, B., K. Spitznogle, and A. Beverfjord. "Attitudes and Use of Pornography in the Norwegian Population 2002," *Journal of Sex Research*, 2004; 41(2):193–200.
4. Ibid.
5. http://advocatesforyouth.org/publications.
6. Mercer, C. H., C. Tanton, P. Prah, B. Erens, P. Sonnenberg, S. Clifton, et al. "Changes in Sexual Attitudes and Lifestyles in Britain through the Life Course and Over Time: Findings from the National Surveys of Sexual Attitudes and Lifestyles (Natsal)," *Lancet*, 2013; 382(9907):1781–94.
7. Marston, C. and R. Lewis. "Anal Heterosex Among Young People and Implications for Health Promotion: A Qualitative Study in the UK," *BMJ open*, 2014; 4(8):e004996.
8. Christopher, F. S. and S. Sprecher. "Sexuality in Marriage, Dating, and Other Relationships: A Decade Review," *Journal of Marriage and Family*, 2000; 62(4): 999–1017.
9. Bernard, M. L. R. "How Often Do Queer Women Have Sex?," *Autostraddle*, 2015; [updated 03/30/2015]. Available at: http://autostraddle.com/how-often-do -lesbians-have-sex-283731/.
10. Stabell, K., B. Mortensen, and B. Træen. "Samleiefrekvens: Prevalens og prediktorer i et tilfeldig utvalg norske gifte og samboende heteroseksuelle par," *Journal of the Norwegian Psychological Association*, 2008; 45:683–94.
11. Klussman, D. "Sexual Motivation and the Duration of Partnership," *Archives of Sexual Behavior*, 2002; 31(3):275–87.
12. Murray, S. H. and R. R. Milhausen. "Sexual Desire and Relationship Duration in Young Men and Women," *Journal of Sex & Marital Therapy*, 2012; 38(1):28–40.
13. Rao, K. V. and A. Demaris. "Coital Frequency Among Married and Cohabiting Couples in the United States," *Journal of Biosocial Science*, 1995; 27(2):135–50.
14. Bernard. "How Often Do Queer Women Have Sex?"
15. Stabell, Mortensen, and Træen. "Samleiefrekvens."

16. Muise, A., U. Schimmack, and E. A. Impett, "Sexual Frequency Predicts Greater Well-Being, But More Is Not Always Better," *Social Psychological and Personality Science*, 2016; 7(4):295–302.

17. Christopher and Sprecher. "Sexuality in Marriage."

18. Sprecher, S. "Sexual Satisfaction in Premarital Relationships: Associations with Satisfaction, Love, Commitment, and Stability," *Journal of Sex Research*, 2002; 39(3):190–6.

19. Haavio-Mannila, E. and O. Kontula. "Correlates of Increased Sexual Satisfaction," *Archives of Sexual Behavior*, 1997; 26(4):399–419.

20. Frederick, A., J. Lever, B. J. Gillespie, and J. R. Garcia. "What Keeps Passion Alive? Sexual Satisfaction Is Associated with Sexual Communication, Mood Setting, Sexual Variety, Oral Sex, Orgasm and Sex Frequency in a National U.S. Study," *Journal of Sex Research*, 2016:1–16.

21. MacNeil, S. and E. S. Byers. "Dyadic Assessment of Sexual Self-Disclosure and Sexual Satisfaction in Heterosexual Dating Couples," *Journal of Social and Personal Relationships*, 2005; 22(2):169–81.

22. Montesi, J. L., R. L. Fauber, E. A. Gordon, and R. G. Heimberg. "The Specific Importance of Communicating About Sex to Couples' Sexual and Overall Relationship Satisfaction," *Journal of Social and Personal Relationships*, 2011; 28(5):591–609.

23. Klussman. "Sexual Motivation."

24. Richters, J., R. Visser, C. Rissel and A. Smith. "Sexual Practices at Last Heterosexual Encounter and Occurrence of Orgasm in a National Survey," *Journal of Sex Research*, 2006; 43(3):217–26.

25. Mitchell, K. R., C. H. Mercer, G. B. Ploubidis, K. G. Jones, J. Datta, N. Field, et al. "Sexual Function in Britain: Findings from the Third National Survey of Sexual Attitudes and Lifestyles (Natsal-3)," *Lancet*, 2013; 382(9907):1817–29.

26. Basson, R. "Sexual Desire and Arousal Disorders in Women," *New England Journal of Medicine*, 2006; 354(14):1497–1506.

27. Shifren, J. L. "Sexual Dysfunction in Women: Epidemiology, Risk Factors, and Evaluation," Waltham, MA: *UpToDate*, 2016; [updated 04/04/2016]. Available at: https://uptodate.com/contents/sexual-dysfunction-in-women-epidemiology-risk -factors-and-evaluation.

28. Basson, R., S. Leiblum, L. Brotto, L. Derogatis, J. Fourcroy, K. Fugl-Meyer, et al. "Definitions of Women's Sexual Dysfunction Reconsidered: Advocating Expansion and Revision," *Journal of Psychosomatic Obstetrics and Gynaecology*, 2003; 24(4):212–19.

29. Brotto, L. A., A. J. Petkau, F. Labrie, and R. Basson. "Predictors of Sexual Desire Disorders in Women," *Journal of Sexual Medicine*, 2011; 8(3):742–53.

30. Nagoski, E. *Come as You Are: The Surprising New Science That Will Transform Your Sex Life* (New York: Simon and Schuster, 2015).

31. Ibid.

32. Ibid.

33. Ibid.

34. Roach, M. *Bonk: The Curious Coupling of Science and Sex* (New York: W. W. Norton, 2008).

35. Chivers, M. L., M. C. Seto, M. L. Lalumiere, E. Laan, and T. Grimbos. "Agreement of Self-Reported and Genital Measures of Sexual Arousal in Men and Women: A Meta-analysis," *Archives of Sexual Behavior*, 2010; 39(1):5–56.

36. Ibid.
37. Ibid.
38. Roach. *Bonk*.
39. Basson, R., R. McInnes, M. D. Smith, G. Hodgson, and N. Koppiker. "Efficacy and Safety of Sildenafil Citrate in Women with Sexual Dysfunction Associated with Female Sexual Arousal Disorder," *Journal of Women's Health & Gender-Based Medicine*, 2002; 11(4):367–77.
40. Shifren, J. L. "Sexual Dysfunction in Women: Management," Waltham, MA: *UpToDate*, 2016; [updated 05/19/2016]. Available at: https://www.uptodate.com/contents/sexual-dysfunction-in-women-management.
41. Davis, S., M. A. Papalia, R. J. Norman, S. O'Neill, M. Redelman, M. Williamson, et al. "Safety and Efficacy of a Testosterone Metered-Dose Transdermal Spray for Treating Decreased Sexual Satisfaction in Premenopausal Women: A Randomized Trial," *Annals of Internal Medicine*, 2008; 148(8):569–77.
42. Ibid.
43. Brotto, Petkau, Labrie, and Basson. "Predictors of Sexual Desire."
44. Clayton, A. H., S. E. Althof, S. Kingsberg, L. R. DeRogatis, R. Kroll, I. Goldstein, et al. "Bremelanotide for Female Sexual Dysfunctions in Premenopausal Women: A Randomized Placebo-Controlled Dose-Finding Trial," *Women's Health*, 2016; 12(3):325–37.
45. http://www.npr.org/sections/health-shots/2015/08/18/432704214/addyi-fda-approves-drug-to-boost-womens-desire.
46. Ibid.
47. Shifren. "Sexual Dysfunction in Women."
48. Bradford, A., C. Meston. "Correlates of Placebo Response in the Treatment of Sexual Dysfunction in Women: A Preliminary Report," *Journal of Sexual Medicine*, 2007; 4(5):1345–51.
49. Nagoski. *Come as You Are*.
50. Meston, C. M., R. J. Levin, M. L. Sipski, E. M. Hull and J. R. Heiman. "Women's Orgasm," *Annual Review of Sex Research*, 2004; 15:173–257.
51. Mah, K. and Y. M. Binik. "The Nature of Human Orgasm: A Critical Review of Major Trends," *Clinical Psychology Review*, 2001; 21(6):823–56.
52. Nagoski. *Come as You Are*.
53. Mah and Binik. "The Nature of Human Orgasm."
54. Wikipedia. "Masturbate-a-thon," *Wikipedia*, 2016; [updated 09/08/2016]. Available at: https://en.wikipedia.org/wiki/Masturbate-a-thon.
55. Puppo, V. "Embryology and Anatomy of the Vulva: The Female Orgasm and Women's Sexual Health," *European Journal of Obstetrics and Gynecology and Reproductive Biology*, 2011; 154(1):3–8.
56. Wallen, K. and E. A. Lloyd. "Female Sexual Arousal: Genital Anatomy and Orgasm in Intercourse," *Hormones and Behavior*, 2011; 59(5):780–92.
57. Korda, J. B., S. W. Goldstein, and F. Sommer. "Sexual Medicine History: The History of Female Ejaculation," *Journal of Sexual Medicine*, 2010; 7(5):1965–75.
58. Rosen, R. "No Female Ejaculation, Please, We're British: A History of Porn and Censorship," *Independent*, 2014; [updated 12/04/2014]. Available at: http://www.independent.co.uk/life-style/health-and-families/features/no-female-ejaculation-please-we-re-british-a-history-of-porn-and-censorship-9903054.html.

59. Pollen, J. J. and A. Dreilinger. "Immunohistochemical Identification of Prostatic Acid Phosphatase and Prostate Specific Antigen in Female Periurethral Glands," *Urology*, 1984; 23(3):303–4.

60. Wimpissinger, F., K. Stifter, W. Grin, and W. Stackl. "The Female Prostate Revisited: Perineal Ultrasound and Biochemical Studies of Female Ejaculate," *Journal of Sexual Medicine*, 2007; 4(5):1388–93.

61. Ibid.

62. Salama, S., F. Boitrelle, A. Gauquelin, L. Malagrida, N. Thiounn, and P. Desvaux. "Nature and Origin of 'Squirting' in Female Sexuality," *Journal of Sexual Medicine*, 2015; 12(3):661–6.

63. Pastor, Z. "Female Ejaculation Orgasm vs. Coital Incontinence: A Systematic Review," *Journal of Sexual Medicine*, 2013; 10(7):1682–91.

64. Laqueur, T. *Making Sex: Body and Gender from the Greeks to Freud* (Boston, MA: Harvard University Press, 1992).

65. Ibid.

66. Freud, S. *Three Essays on the Theory of Sexuality* (1905).

67. Levin, R. J. "Recreation and Procreation: A Critical View of Sex in the Human Female," *Clinical Anatomy*, 2015; 28(3):339–54.

68. Angel, K. "The History of 'Female Sexual Dysfunction' as a Mental Disorder in the 20th Century," *Current Opinion in Psychiatry*, 2010; 23(6):536.

69. Roach. *Bonk*.

70. Wallen and Lloyd. "Female Sexual Arousal."

71. Oakley, S. H., C. M. Vaccaro, C. C. Crisp, M. Estanol, A. N. Fellner, S. D. Kleeman, et al. "Clitoral Size and Location in Relation to Sexual Function Using Pelvic MRI," *Journal of Sexual Medicine*, 2014; 11(4):1013–22.

72. Strömqvist, L. "Kunskapens frukt," *Galago*, 2014.

73. Nagoski. *Come as You Are*.

74. Mitchell, Mercer, Ploubidis, Jones, Datta, Field, et al. "Sexual Function in Britain."

75. Dunn, K. M., L. F. Cherkas, and T. D. Spector. "Genetic Influences on Variation in Female Orgasmic Function: A Twin Study," *Biology Letters*, 2005; 1(3):260–3.

76. Dawood, K., K. M. Kirk, J. M. Bailey, P. W. Andrews, and N. G. Martin. "Genetic and Environmental Influences on the Frequency of Orgasm in Women," *Twin Research and Human Genetics*, 2005; 8(1):27–33.

77. Armstrong, E. A., P. England, and A. C. Fogarty. "Accounting for Women's Orgasm and Sexual Enjoyment in College Hookups and Relationships," *American Sociological Review*, 2012; 77(3):435–62.

78. Kohlenberg, R. J. "Directed Masturbation and the Treatment of Primary Orgasmic Dysfunction," *Archives of Sexual Behavior*, 1974; 3(4):349–56.

79. Bradford, A. "Treatment of Female Orgasmic Disorder," Waltham, MA: *UpToDate*, 2016; Available at: https://uptodate.com/contents/treatment-of-female-orgasmic-disorder.

80. Eichel, E. W., J. D. Eichel, and S. Kule. "The Technique of Coital Alignment and Its Relation to Female Orgasmic Response and Simultaneous Orgasm," *Journal of Sex & Marital Therapy*, 1988; 14(2):129–41.

81. Pierce, A. P. "The Coital Alignment Technique (CAT): An Overview of Studies," *Journal of Sex & Marital Therapy*, 2000; 26(3):257–68.

82. Rosenbaum, T. Y. "Reviews: Pelvic Floor Involvement in Male and Female Sexual Dysfunction and the Role of Pelvic Floor Rehabilitation in Treatment: A Literature Review," *Journal of Sexual Medicine*, 2007; 4(1):4–13.
83. Lorenz, T. A. and C. M. Meston. "Exercise Improves Sexual Function in Women Taking Antidepressants: Results from a Randomized Crossover Trial," *Depression and Anxiety*, 2014; 31(3):188–95.
84. Roach. *Bonk*.

CONTRACEPTION

1. http://www.pbs.org/wnet/need-to-know/health/a-brief-history-of-the-birth-control-pill/480/.
2. Johansen, M. "P-piller," *Emetodebok for seksuell helse* (Oslo: Sex og samfunn, 2016).
3. Johansen, M. "P-ring," *Emetodebok for seksuell helse* (Oslo: Sex og samfunn, 2016).
4. Johansen, M. "P-plaster," *Emetodebok for seksuell helse* (Oslo: Sex og samfunn, 2016).
5. Johansen, M. "P-stav," *Emetodebok for seksuell helse* (Oslo: Sex og samfunn, 2016).
6. Johansen, M. "Hormon-spiral," *Emetodebok for seksuell helse* (Oslo: Sex og samfunn, 2016).
7. Johansen, M. "Gestagen p-piller," *Emetodebok for seksuell helse* (Oslo: Sex og samfunn, 2016).
8. Johansen, M. "Minipiller," *Emetodebok for seksuell helse* (Oslo: Sex og samfunn, 2016).
9. Johansen, M. "P-sprøyte," *Emetodebok for seksuell helse* (Oslo: Sex og samfunn, 2016).
10. https://www.plannedparenthood.org/learn/birth-control/female-condom/how-do-i-use-a-female-condom.
11. Jennings, V. "Fertility Awareness-Based Methods of Pregnancy Prevention," Waltham, MA: *UpToDate*, 2016. Available at: https://www.uptodate.com/contents/fertility-awareness-based-methods-of-pregnancy-prevention.
12. http://plannedparenthood.tumblr.com/post/28521852221/how-much-does-an-iud-cost.
13. Dean, G. and A. B. Goldberg. "Intrauterine Contraception: Devices, Candidates, and Selection," Waltham, MA: *UpToDate*, 2016; [updated 09/15/2016]. Available at: https://www.uptodate.com/contents/intrauterine-contraception-devices-candidates-and-selection.
14. Nesheim, B. I. "Prevensjon," in *Obstetrikk og gynekologi*, ed. J. M. Maltau, K. Molne, B. I. Nesheim, 3rd ed. (Oslo: Gyldendal Akademisk, 2015), 313–14.
15. Ibid.
16. http://americansocietyforec.org.
17. Johansen, M. "Nødprevensjon: Levonorgestrel," *Emetodebok for seksuell helse* (Oslo: Sex og samfunn, 2016).
18. http://www.ellanow.com.
19. Bordvik, M. "P-pille-bruk kan ødelegge effekten av angrepille," *Dagens Medisin*, 2016; [updated 06/07/2016]. Available at: http://www.dagensmedisin.no/artikler/2016/07/06/angrepille-kan-odelegge-p-pille-effekt/.
20. Johansen, M. "Nødprevensjon: Ulipristalacetat," *Emetodebok for seksuell helse* (Oslo: *Sex og samfunn*, 2016).
21. Johansen. "Kobberspiral."
22. World Health Organization. "Family Planning/Contraception," *WHO*, 2016.

23. Johansen, M. "Prevensjonsmidler," *Emetodebok for seksuell helse* (Oslo: Sex og samfunn, 2016).
24. http://www.who.int/mediacentre/factsheets/fs351/en/.
25. Nesheim. "Prevensjon."
26. Juvkam, K. H., and H. B. Gudim. "Medikamentell forskyvning av menstruasjon," *Tidsskrift for Den norske legeforening*, 2013; 133:166–68.
27. Legemiddelhåndboken. "Perorale gestagener," *Norsk Legemiddelhåndbok*, 2016; [updated 09/13/2016]. Available at: http://legemiddelhandboka.no/legemidler/?frid=lk-03-endokr-7205.
28. Rosenberg, M. J., and M. S. Waugh. "Oral Contraceptive Discontinuation: A Prospective Evaluation of Frequency and Reasons," *American Journal of Obstetrics and Gynecology*, 1998; 179(3):577–82.
29. Ibid.
30. Barsky, A. J., R. Saintfort, M. P. Rogers, and J. F. Borus. "Non-specific Medication Side Effects and the Nocebo Phenomenon," *JAMA*, 2002; 287(5):622–7.
31. Peipert, J. F., and J. Gutmann. "Oral Contraceptive Risk Assessment: A Survey of 247 Educated Women," *Obstetrics & Gynecology*, 1993; 82(1):112–17.
32. Grimes, D. A. and K. F. Schulz. "Nonspecific Side Effects of All Contraceptives: Nocebo or Noise?," *Contraception*, 2011; 83(1):5–9.
33. Johansen. "Prevensjonsmidler."
34. Martin, K. A. and P. S. Douglas. "Risk and Side Effects Associated with Estrogen-Progestin Contraceptives," Waltham, MA: *UpToDate*, 2016; [updated 08/22/2016]. Available at: https//www.uptodate.com/contents/risks-and-side-effects-associated-with-estrogen-progestin-contraceptives.
35. NEL—Norsk elektronisk legehåndbok. "Melasma," *NEL*, 2015; [updated 12/28/2015]. Available at: https://legehandboka.no/handboken/kliniske-kapitler/hud/tilstander-og-sykdommer/pitmenterte-lesjoner/melasma-kloasma/.
36. Gallo, M. F., D. A. Grimes, K. F. Schulz, and F. M. Helmerhorst. "Combination Estrogen-Progestin Contraceptives and Body Weight: Systematic Review of Randomized Controlled Trials," *Obstetrics & Gynecology*, 2004; 103(2):359–73.
37. Moen, M. H. "Selvvalgt menstruasjon," *Tidsskrift for Den norsk legeforening*, 2013; 133:131.
38. Johansen. "Hormon-spiral."
39. Charlton, B. M., J. W. Rich-Edwards, G. A. Colditz, S. A. Missmer, B. A. Rosner, S. E. Hankinson, et al. "Oral Contraceptive Use and Mortality after 36 Years of Follow-Up in the Nurses' Health Study: Prospective Cohort Study," *BMJ*, 2014; 349:g6356.
40. Kaunitz, A. M. "Patient Education: Hormonal Methods of Birth Control (Beyond the Basics)," Walton, MA: *UpToDate*, 2016. Available at: https://www.uptodate.com/contents/hormonal-methods-of-birth-control-beyond-the-basics?source=see_link.
41. Heit, J. A., C. E. Kobbervig, A. H. James, T. M. Petterson, K. R. Bailey, and L. J. Melton. "Trends in the Incidence of Venous Thromboembolism during Pregnancy or Postpartum: A 30-Year Population-Based Study," *Annals of Internal Medicine*, 2005; 143(10):697–706.
42. Lidegaard, O., E. Lokkegaard, A. Jensen, C. W. Skovlund, and N. Keiding. "Thrombotic Stroke and Myocardial Infarction with Hormonal Contraception," *New England Journal of Medicine*, 2012; 366(24):2257–66.

43. Martin, and Douglas. "Risk and Side Effects."
44. Hannaford, P. C., S. Selvaraj, A. M. Elliott, V. Angus, L. Iversen, and A. J. Lee. "Cohort Data from the Royal College of General Practitioners' Oral Contraception Study," *BMJ*, 2007; 335(7621):651.
45. Martin and Douglas. "Risk and Side Effects."
46. Beral, V., R. Doll, C. Hermon, R. Peto, and G. Reeves. "Ovarian Cancer and Oral Contraceptives: Collaborative Reanalysis of Data from 45 Epidemiological Studies including 23,257 Women with Ovarian Cancer 87,303 Controls," *Lancet*, 2008; 371(9609):303–14.
47. Vessey, M. and R. Painter. "Oral Contraceptive Use and Cancer. Findings in a Large Cohort Study, 1968–2004," *British Journal of Cancer*, 2006; 95:385–9.
48. Appleby, P., V. Beral, A. Berrington de Gonzalez, D. Colin, S. Franceschi, A. Goodhill, et al. "Cervical Cancer and Hormonal Contraceptives: Collaborative Reanalysis of Individual Data for 16,573 Women with Cervical Cancer and 35,509 Women without Cervical Cancer from 24 Epidemiological Studies," *Lancet*, 2007; 370(9599):1609–21.
49. Martin and Douglas. "Risk and Side Effects."
50. Stanislaw, H. and F. J. Rice. "Correlation between Sexual Desire and Menstrual Cycle Characteristics," *Archives of Sexual Behaviour*, 1988; 17(6):499–508.
51. Caruso, S., C. Agnello, C. Malandrino, L. Lo Presti, C. Cicero, and S. Cianci. "Do Hormones Influence Women's Sex? Sexual Activity over the Menstrual Cycle," *Journal of Sexual Medicine*, 2014; 11(1):211–21.
52. Bellis, M. A. and R. R. Baker. "Do Females Promote Sperm Competition? Data for Humans," *Animal Behaviour*, 1990; 40(5):997–9.
53. Grimes and Schulz. "Nonspecific Side Effects."
54. Lindh, I. and F. Blohm, A. Andersson-Ellstrom, and I. Milsom. "Contraceptive Use and Pregnancy Outcome in Three Generations of Swedish Female Teenagers from the Same Urban Population," *Contraception*, 2009; 80(2):163–9.
55. Brunner Huber, I. R., C. J. Hogue, A. D. Stein, C. Drews, M. Zieman, J. King, et al. "Contraceptive Use and Discontinuation: Findings from the Contraceptive History, Initiation, and Choice Study," *American Journal of Obstetrics and Gynecology*, 2006; 194(5):1290–5.
56. Martin and Douglas. "Risk and Side Effects."
57. O'Connell, K., A. R. Davis, and J. Kerns. "Oral Contraceptives: Side Effects and Depression in Adolescent Girls," *Contraception*, 2007; 75(4):299–304.
58. Redmond, G., A. J. Godwin, W. Olson, and J. S. Lippman. "Use of Placebo Controls in an Oral Contraceptive Trial: Methodological Issues and Adverse Event Incidence," *Contraception*, 1999; 60(2):81–85.
59. Graham, C. A., and B. B. Sherwin. "The Relationship between Mood and Sexuality in Women Using an Oral Contraceptive as a Treatment for Premenstrual Symptoms," *Psychoneuroendocrinology*, 1993; 18(4):273–81.
60. Graham, C. A., R. Ramos, J. Bancroft, C. Maglaya, and T. M. Farley. "The Effects of Steroid Contraceptives on the Well-Being and Sexuality of Women: A Double-Blind, Placebo-Controlled, Two-Centre Study of Combined and Progestogen-Only Methods," *Contraception*, 1995; 52(6):363–9.
61. Gingnell, M., J. Engman, A. Frick, L. Moby, J. Wikstrom, M. Fredrikson, et al. "Oral Contraceptive Use Changes in Brain Activity and Mood in Women with Previous Negative Affect on the Pill—a Double-Blinded, Placebo-Controlled

Randomized Trial of a Levonorgestrel-Containing Combined Oral Contraceptive," *Psychoneuroendocrinology*, 2013; 38(7):1133–44.

62. Jacobi, F., H. U. Wittchen, C. Holting, M. Hofler, H. Pfister, N. Muller, et al. "Prevalence, Co-Morbidity and Correlates of Mental Disorders in the General Population: Results from the German Health Interview and Examination Survey (GHS)," *Psychological Medicine*, 2004; 34(4):597–611.

63. Joffe, H., L. S. Cohen, and B. L. Harlow. "Impact of Oral Contraceptive Pill Use on Premenstrual Mood: Predictors of Improvement and Deterioration," *American Journal of Obstetrics and Gynecology*, 2003; 189(6):1523–30.

64. Duke, J. M., D. W. Sibbritt, and A. F. Young. "Is There an Association Between the Use of Oral Contraception and Depressive Symptoms in Young Australian Women?," *Contraception*, 2007; 75(1):27–31.

65. Keyes, K. M., K. Cheslack-Postava, C. Westhoff, C. M. Heim, M. Haloosim, K. Walsh, et al. "Association of Hormonal Contraceptive Use with Reduced Levels of Depressive Symptoms: National Study of Sexually Active Women in the United States," *American Journal of Epidemiology*, 2013; 178(9):1378–88.

66. Toffol, E., O. Heikinheimo, P. Koponen, R. Luoto, and T. Partonen. "Hormonal Contraception and Mental Health: Results of a Population-Based Study," *Human Reproduction*, 2011; 26(11):3085–93.

67. Skovlund, C., L. Mørch, L. Kessing, and Ø. Lidegaard. "Association of Hormonal Contraception with Depression," *JAMA Psychiatry*, 2016; 73(11):1154–62.

68. Malmborg, A., E. Persson, J. Brynhildsen, and M. Hammar. "Hormonal Contraception and Sexual Desire: A Questionnaire-Based Study of Young Swedish Women," *European Journal of Contraception & Reproductive Healthcare*, 2016; 21(2):158–67.

69. Pastor, Z., K. Holla, and R. Chmel. "The Influence of Combined Oral Contraceptives on Female Sexual Desire: A Systematic Review," *European Journal of Contraception & Reproductive Healthcare*, 2013; 18(1):27–43.

70. Davis, Papalia, Norman, O'Neill, Redelman, Williamson, et al. "Safety and Efficacy."

71. Burrows, L. J., M. Basha, and A. T. Goldstein. "The Effects of Hormonal Contraceptives on Female Sexuality: A Review," *Journal of Sexual Medicine*, 2012; 9(9):2213–23.

72. Cheung, E., and C. Free. "Factors Influencing Young Women's Decision Making regarding Hormonal Contraceptives: A Qualitative Study," *Contraception*, 2004; 71(6):426–31.

73. Lidegaard, O., E. Lokkegaard, A. L. Svendsen, and C. Agger. "Hormonal Contraception and Risk of Venous Thromboembolism: National Follow-Up Study," *BMJ*, 2009; 339:b2890.

74. Johansen, M. "Misoppfatninger om prevensjon," *Emetodebok for seksuell helse* (Oslo: Sex og samfunn, 2016).

75. Bagwell, M. A., S. J. Thompson, C. L. Addy, A. L. Coker, and E. R. Baker. "Primary Infertility and Oral Contraceptive Steroid Use," *Fertility and Sterility*, 1995; 63(6):1161–6.

76. Mansour, D., K. Gemzell-Danielsson, P. Inki, and J. T. Jensen. "Fertility after Discontinuation of Contraception: A Comprehensive Review of the Literature," *Contraception*, 2011; 845(5):465–77.

ABORTION

1. http://www.businessinsider.com/how-many-abortion-clinics-are-in-america -each-state-2017-2.
2. http://www.thelancet.com/journals/lancet/article/PIIS0140-6736(16)30380-4/ abstract.
3. UNDP/UNFPA/WHO/World Bank Special Programme of Research, Development and Research Training in Human Reproduction (HRP). "Unsafe Abortion Incidence and Mortality—Global and Regional Levels in 2008 and Trends," *WHO*, 2012.
4. Singh, S. and I. Maddow-Zimet. "Facility-Based Treatment for Medical Complications Resulting from Unsafe Pregnancy Termination in the Developing World, 2012: A Review of Evidence from 26 Countries," *BJOG*, 2016; 123:1489–98.
5. Bjørge, L., M. Løkeland, and K. S. Oppegaard. "Provosert abort," *Veileder i gynekologi 2015*, Norsk gynekologisk forening, 2015.
6. Cedars, M. I. and Y. Anaya. "Intrauterine Adhesions," Waltham, MA: *UpToDate*, 2016; [updated 06/03/2016]. Available at: https://www.uptodate.com/contents/ uterine-adhesions.

TROUBLE DOWN BELOW

1. NEL—Norsk elektronisk legehåndbok. "Sekundær amenoré," *NEL*, 2014; [updated 07/21/2014]. Available at: https:///legehandboka.no/handboken/kliniske-kapitler -gynekologi/symptomer-og-tegn/amenore-sekundar-/.
2. Ibid.
3. Dawood, M. Y. "Primary Dysmenorrhea: Advances in Pathogenesis and Management," *Obstetrics & Gynecology*, 2006; 108(2):428–41.
4. Ibid.
5. Ibid.
6. Rapkin, A. J., et al. "Pelvic Pain and Dysmenorrhea," in *Berek and Novak's Gynecology*, ed. J. S. Berek, 15th ed. (Philadelphia, PA: Lippincott Williams and Wilkins, 2012), 482.
7. Johansen, M. "Menstruasjon," *Emetodebok for seksuell helse* (Oslo: Sex og samfunn, 2016).
8. Ibid.
9. Rapkin et al. "Pelvic Pain and Dysmenorrhea," 485.
10. Hornstein, M. D. and W. E. Gibbons. "Pathogenesis and Treatment of Infertility in Women with Endometriosis," Waltham, MA: *UpToDate*, 2016; [updated 10/10/2013]. Available at: https://www.uptodate.com/contents/treatment-of -infertility-in-women-with-endometriosis.
11. Kisic, J., H. K. Opøien, I. M. Ringen, A. Veddeng, A. Langebrekke. "Endometriose," *Veileder i Gynekologi 2015*, Norsk gynekologisk forening, 2015.
12. Rapkin, et al. "Pelvic Pain and Dysmenorrhea," 485.
13. Wilson, E. E. "Polycystic Ovarian Syndrome and Hyperandrogenism," in *Williams Gynecology*, ed. B. L. Hoffman, J. O. Schorge, J. I. Schaffer, L. M. Halvorsen, K. D. Bradshaw, F. G. Cunningham, 2nd ed. (New York: McGraw Hill Medical, 2012).
14. Goodarzi, M. O. "Polycystic Ovary Syndrome. Best Practice," *BMJ*, 2016; [updated 06/20/2016]. Available at: http://bestpractice.bmj.com/best-practice-monograph/ 141/follow-up/complications.html.

15. Legro, R. S., H. X. Barnhart, W. D. Schlaff, B. R. Carr, M. P. Diamond, S. A. Carson, et al. "Clomiphene, Metforin, or Both for Infertility in the Polycystic Ovary Syndrome," *New England Journal of Medicine*, 2007; 356(6):551–66.
16. Hardiman, P., O. S. Pillay, and W. Atiomo. "Polycystic Ovary Syndrome and Endometrial Carcinoma," *Lancet*, 2003; 361(9371):1810–12.
17. Haoula, Z., M. Salman, and W. Atiomo. "Evaluating the Association between Endometrial Cancer and Polycystic Ovary Syndrome," *Human Reproduction*, 2012; 27(5):1327–31.
18. Goodarzi, "Polycystic Ovary Syndrome."
19. Ibid.
20. Wilson. "Polycystic Ovarian Syndrome."
21. Goodarzi, "Polycystic Ovary Syndrome."
22. Ibid.
23. Heinzman, A. B. and B. L. Hoffman. "Pelvic Mass," in *Williams Gynecology*, ed. B. L. Hoffman, J. O. Schorge, J. L. Schaffer, L. M. Halvorsen, K. D. Bradshaw, F. G. Cunningham, 2nd ed. (New York: McGraw Hill Medical, 2012).
24. Ibid.
25. Klatsky, P. C., N. D. Tran, A. B. Caughey, and V. Y. Fujimoto. "Fibroids and Reproductive Outcomes: A Systematic Literature Review from Conception to Delivery," *American Journal of Obstetrics and Gynecology*, 2008; 198(4):357–66.
26. Tulandi, T. "Reproductive Issues in Women with Uterine Leiomyomas (Fibroids)," Waltham, MA: *UpToDate*, 2016; [updated 11/24/2015]. Available at: https://www.uptodate.com/contents/reproductive-issues-in-women-with-uterine-leiomyomas-fibroids.
27. Pritts, E. A., W. H. Parker, D. L. Olive. "Fibroids and Infertility: An Updated Systematic Review of the Evidence," *Fertility and Sterility*, 2009; 91(4):1215–23.
28. Ibid.
29. Klatsky, Tran, Caughey, and Fujimoto. "Fibroids and Reproductive Outcomes."
30. Tulandi. "Reproductive Issues in Women."
31. Stewart, E. A. "Epidemiology, Clinical Manifestations, Diagnosis, and Natural History of Uterine Leiomyomas (Fibroids)," Waltham MA: *UpToDate*, 2016; [updated 05/29/2015]. Available at: https://www.uptodate.com/contents/epidemiology-clinical-manifestations-diagnosis-and-natural-history-of-uterine-leiomyomas-fibroids.
32. Ibid.
33. Stewart, E. G. "Clinical Manifestations and Diagnosis of Generalized Vulvodynia," Waltham MA: *UpToDate*, 2016; [updated 01/30/2015]. Available at: https://www.uptodate.com/contents/clinical-manifestations-and-diagnosis-of-generalized-vulvodynia.
34. Iglesia, C. "Clinical Manifestations and Diagnosis of Localized Vulvar Pain Syndrome (Formerly Vulvodynia, Vestibulodynia, Vulvar Vestibulitis, or Focal Vulvitis)," Waltham MA: *UpToDate*, 2016; [updated 05/25/2015]. Available at: https://www.uptodate.com/contents/clinical-manifestations-and-diagnosis-of-localized-vulvar-pain-syndrome-formerly-vulvodynia-vestibulitis-or-focal-vulvitis.
35. Johansen, M. "Vanlige sexologiske problemer hos kvinner," *Emetodebok for seksuell helse* (Oslo: Sex og samfunn, 2016).
36. Farmer, M. A., A. M. Taylor, A. L. Bailey, A. H. Tuttle, L. C. MacIntyre, Z. E. Milagrosa, et al. "Repeated Vulvovaginal Fungal Infections Cause Persistent Pain in a Mouse Model of Vulvodynia," *Science Translational Medicine*, 2011; 3(101):10191.

294   Notes

37. Helgesen, A. L. "Når samleiet gjør vondt," *Forskning.no*, 2015; [updated 05/15/2015]. Available at: http://forskning.no/blogg/kvinnehelsebloggen/nar-samleiet-gjor -vondt.
38. Tympanidis, P., M. Casula, Y. Yiangou, G. Terenghi, P. Dowd, and P. Anand. "Increased Vanilloid Receptor VRI Innervation in Vulvodynia," *European Journal of Pain*, 2004; 8(2):129–33.
39. Tympanidis, P., G. Terenghi, and P. Dowd. "Increased Innervation of the Vulval Vestibule in Patients with Vulvodynia," *British Journal of Dermatology*, 2003; 148(5):1021–7.
40. Khandker, M., S. S. Brady, A. F. Vitonis, R. F. Maclehose, E. G. Stewart, and B. L. Harlow. "The Influence of Depression and Anxiety on Risk of Adult Onset Vulvodynia," *Journal of Women's Health*, 2011; 20(10):1445–51.
41. Reed, B. D., H. K. Haefner, M. R. Punch, R. S. Roth, D. W. Gorenflo, and B. W. Gillespie. "Psychosocial and Sexual Functioning in Women with Vulvodynia and Chronic Pelvic Pain. A Comparative Evaluation," *Journal of Reproductive Medicine*, 2000; 45(8):624–32.
42. For more information and a list of vulvodynia treatment providers in the United States, see https://www.nva.org/for-patients/health-care-provider-list/.
43. NEL—Norsk elektronisk legehåndbok. "Smerte og ubehag i vulva," *NEL*, 2015. Available at: https://legehandboka.no/handboken/kliniske-kapitler/gynekologi/ symptomer-og-tegn/smerte-og-ubehag-i-vulva/.
44. Stewart, E. G. "Differential Diagnosis of Sexual Pain in Women," Waltham, MA: *UpToDate*, 2016; [updated 11/18/2015]. Available at: https://www.uptodate.com/ contents/differential-diagnosis-of-sexual-pain-in-women.
45. Ibid.
46. Bjørnstad, S. "Jeg bruker aldri kondom, jeg ser om jenter har en kjønnssykdom," Page 2, 2015; [updated 03/09/2015]. Available at: http://www.side2 .no/underholdning/-jeg-bruker-aldri-kondom-jeg-ser-om-jenter-har-en -kjnnssykdom/8551263.html.
47. http://www.factlv.org/timeline.htm.
48. UNAIDS. "Fact Sheet 2016," UNAIDS, 2016.
49. https://www.cdc.gov/hiv/statistics/overview/ataglance.html.
50. Moi, H. and J. M. Maltau. *Seksuelt overførbare infeksjoner og genitale hudsykdommer*. 3rd ed. (Oslo: Gyldendal Akademisk, 2013).
51. NEL—Norsk elektronisk legehåndbok. "Genital klamydiainfeksjon hos kvinner," *NEL*, 2016. Available at: https://legehandboka.no/handboken/kliniske-kapitler/ gynekologi/tilstander-og-sykdommer/infeksjoner/klamydiainfeksjon-hos-kvinner/.
52. Jensen, J. S., M. Cusini, M. Gomberg, and H. Moi. "2016 European Guideline on Mycoplasma genitalium Infections," *Journal of the European Academy of Dermatology and Venereology*, 2016.
53. Ross, J. "Pelvic Inflammatory Disease: Pathogenesis, Microbiology, and Risk Factors," Waltham, MA: *UpToDate*, 2016; [updated 02/19/2015]. Available at: https://www.uptodate.com/contents/pelvic-inflammatory-disease-pathogenesis -microbiology-and-risk-factors.
54. Sweet, R. L. "Pelvic Inflammatory Disease: Current Concepts of Diagnosis and Management," *Current Infectious Disease Reports*, 2012; 14(2):194–203.
55. Johansen, M. "Infeksjoner," *Emetodebok for seksuell helse* (Oslo: Sex og samfunn, 2016).

56. https://www.cdc.gov/std.
57. Moi and Maltau. *Seksuelt overførbare infeksjoner.*
58. Chayavichitsilp, P., J. V. Buckwalter, A. C. Krakowski, and S. F. Friedlander. "Herpes Simplex," *Pediatr Rev*, 2009; 30(4):119–29; quiz 130.
59. Ibid.
60. Ibid.
61. Ibid.
62. Ibid.
63. Ibid.
64. Sobel, J. D. "Candida Vulvovaginitis," Waltham, MA: *UpToDate*, 2016. Available at: https://www.uptodate.com/contents/candida-vulvovaginitis.
65. NEL—Norsk elektronisk legehåndbok. "Candida vaginitt," *NEL*, 2016; [updated 02/02/2016]. Available at: https://legehandboka.no/handboken/kliniske-kapitler/gynekologi/tilstander-og-sykdommer/infeksjoner/candida-vaginitt/.
66. Friedman, M. "This Woman Is Making Sourdough Bread Using Yeast from Her Vagina," *Cosmopolitan*, 2015; [updated 11/24/2015]. Available at: http://www.cosmopolitan.com/sex-love/news/a49782/zoe-stavri-sourdough-bread-vagina-yeast/.
67. Sobel. "Candida Vulvovaginitis."
68. Ferris, D. G., P. Nyirjesy, J. D. Sobel, D. Soper, A. Pavletic, and M. S. Litaker. "Over-the-Counter Antifungal Drug Misuse Associated with Patient-Diagnosed Vulvovaginal Candidiasis," *Obstetrics & Gynecology*, 2002; 99(3):419–25.
69. Sobel. "Candida Vulvovaginitis."
70. Lopez, J. E. M. "Candidiasis (Vulvovaginal)," *BMJ—Clinical Evidence*, 2015; [updated 03/16/2015]. Available at: http://clinicalevidence.bmj.com/x/systematic-review/0815/overview.html.
71. Sobel. "Candida Vulvovaginitis."
72. NEL—Norsk elektronisk legehåndbok. "Ukomplisert cystitt hos kvinner," *NEL*, 2016; [updated 07/06/2016]. Available at: https://legehandboka.no/handboken/kliniske-kapitler/nyrer-og-urinveier/tilstander-og-sykdommer/infeksjoner/urinveisinfeksjon-hos-kvinner-ukomplisert/.
73. http://www.clevelandclinicmeded.com/medicalpubs/diseasemanagement/infectious-disease/urinary-tract-infection/.
74. Jepson, R. G., G. Williams, and J. C. Craig. "Cranberries for Preventing Urinary Tract Infections," *Cochrane Library*, 2012.
75. NEL. "Ukomplisert cystitt hos kvinner."
76. Weiss, B. D. "Selecting Medications for the Treatment of Urinary Incontinence," *American Family Physician*, 2005; 71(2):315–22.
77. NEL—Norsk elektronisk legehåndbok. "Stressinkontinens," *NEL*, 2015; [updated 09/08/2015]. Available at: https://legehandboka.no/handboken/kliniske-kapitler/nyrer-og-urinveier/tilstander-og-sykdommer/lekkasjeproblemer/stressinkontinens/.
78. Glazener, C. M., G. P. Herbison, P. D. Wilson, C. MacArthur, G. D. Lang, H. Gee, et al. "Conservative Management of Persistent Postnatal Urinary and Faecal Incontinence: Randomised Controlled Trial," *BMJ*, 2001; 323(7313):593.
79. NEL. "Stressinkontinens."
80. O'Halloran, T., R. J. Bell, P. J. Robinson, and S. R. Davis. "Urinary Incontinence in Young Nulligravid Women: A Cross-Sectional Analysis," *Ann Intern Med*, 2012; 157(2):87–93.

81. Simeonova, Z., I. Milsom, A. M. Kullendorff, U. Molander, and C. Bengtsson. "The Prevalence of Urinary Incontinence and Its Influence on the Quality of Life in Women from an Urban Swedish Population," *Acta Obstetricia et Gynecologica Scandinavica*, 1999; 78(6):546–51.
82. NEL. "Stressinkontinens."
83. NEL—Norsk elektronisk legehåndbok. "Urgeinkontinens hos kvinner," *NEL*, 2016; [updated 03/07/2016]. Available at: https://legehandboka.no/handboken/kliniske-kapitler/nyrer-og-urinveier/tilstander-og-sykdommer/lekkasjeproblemer/urgeinkontinens-hos-kvinner/.
84. Riss, S., F. A. Weiser, K. Schwameis, T. Riss, M. Mittlbock, G. Steiner, et al. "The Prevalence of Hemorrhoids in Adults," *International Journal of Colorectal Disease*, 2012; 27(2):215–20.
85. Ibid.
86. https://www.cdc.gov/std/stats15/other.htm.
87. Griffith, W. F. and C. L. Werner. "Preinvasive Lesions of the Lower Genital Tract," in *Williams Gynecology*, ed. B. L. Hoffman, J. O. Schorge, J. I. Schaffer, L. M. Halvorsen, K. D. Bradshaw, F. G. Cunningham, 2nd ed. (New York: McGraw Hill Medical, 2012).
88. Östör, A. G. "Natural History of Cervical Intraepithelial Neoplasia: A Critical Review," *International Journal of Gynecological Pathology*, 1993; 12(2):186.
89. https://www.plannedparenthood.org/learn/stds-hiv-safer-sex/hpv/should-i-get-hpv-vaccine.
90. Folkehelseinstituttet. "Vaksinasjonsdekning i prosent (fullvaksinerte) per 12.31.2014 16-åringer (f. 1998)," *FHI*, 2014; 04.23.2014.
91. Statens Serum Institut. "Human papillomavirus-vaccine (HPV) 1, vaccinations-tilslutning," *Statens Serum Institut, Danmark*, 2016.
92. http://www.npr.org/sections/health-shots/2016/08/19/490620216/parents-feel-better-about-hpv-shots-for-teens-if-they-can-opt-out.
93. Statens legemiddelverk. "Meldte mistenkte bivirkninger av HPV-vaksine (Gardasil) —oppdaterte bivirkningstall per 31. desember 2015," *Statens legemiddelverk*, 2016.
94. Feiring, B., et al. "HPV Vaccination and Risk of Chronic Fatigue Syndrome/Myalgic Encephalomyelitis: A Nationwide Register-Based Study from Norway," *Vaccine*, 2017; 35(33):23. Available at: https://doi.org/10.1016/j.vaccine.2017.06.031.
95. European Medicines Agency. "Review Concludes Evidence Does Not Support that HPV Vaccines Cause CRPS or POTS," *European Medicines Agency*, 2015; 11/5/2015.
96. Hviid, A., et al. "Human Papillomavirus Vaccination of Adult Women and Risk of Autoimmune and Neurological Diseases," *J Intern Med*, 2017; DOI: 10.1111/joim.12694.
97. Zuckerberg, M. "Priscilla and I have some exciting news: we're expecting a baby girl!" *Facebook*, 2015; [updated 07/31/2015]. Available at: https://www.facebook.com/photo.php?fbid=10102276573729791&set=a.529237706231.2034669.4&type=1&theater.
98. Hasan, R., D. D. Baird, A. H. Herring, A. F. Olshan, M. L. Jonsson Funk, and K. E. Hartmann. "Patterns and Predictors of Vaginal Bleeding in the First Trimester of Pregnancy," *Annals of Epidemiology*, 2010; 20(7):524–31.
99. Ræder, M. B., A. L. Wollen, R. Braut, and R. Glad. "Spontanabort," *Veileder i Gynekologi 2015*, Norsk gynekologisk forening, 2015.

100. Tulandi, T. and H. M. Al-Fozan. "Spontaneous Abortion: Risk Factors, Etiology, Clinical Manifestations, and Diagnostic Evaluation," Waltham, MA: *UpToDate*, 2016; [updated 11/07/2016]. Available at: https://www.uptodate.com/contents/spontaneous-abortion-risk-factors-etiology-clinical-manifestations-anddiagnostic-evaluation.
101. Ibid.
102. Bardos, J., D. Hercz, J. Friedenthal, S. A. Missmer, and Z. Williams. "A National Survey on Public Perceptions of Miscarriage," *Obstetrics & Gynecology*, 2015; 125(6):1313–20.
103. Nybo Andersen, A. M., J. Wohlfahrt, P. Christens, J. Olsen, and M. Melbye. "Maternal Age and Fetal Loss: Population-Based Register Linkage Study," *BMJ*, 2000; 320(7251):1708–12.
104. Pineles, B. L., E. Park, and J. M. Samet. "Systematic Review and Meta-Analysis of Miscarriage and Maternal Exposure to Tobacco Smoke During Pregnancy," *American Journal of Epidemiology*, 2014; 179(7):807–23.
105. Chatenoud, L., F. Parazzini, E. di Cintio, G. Zanconato, G. Benzi, R. Bortolus, et al. "Paternal and Maternal Smoking Habits Before Conception and During the First Trimester: Relation to Spontaneous Abortion," *Annals of Epidemiology*, 1998; 8(8):520–6.
106. Tulandi and Al-Fozan. "Spontaneous Abortion."
107. Oster, E. *Expecting Better—Why the Conventional Pregnancy Wisdom Is Wrong and What You Really Need to Know* (New York: Penguin Press, 2013).
108. Andersen, A. M. N., P. K. Andersen, J. Olsen, M. Grønbæk, and K. Strandberg-Larsen. "Moderate Alcohol Intake during Pregnancy and Risk of Fetal Death," *International Journal of Epidemiology*, 2012; 41(2):405–13.
109. Nisenblat, V. and R. J. Norman. "The Effects of Caffeine on Reproductive Outcomes in Women," Waltham, MA: *UpToDate*, 2016; [updated 08/24/2016]. Available at: https://www.uptodate.com/contents/the-effects-of-caffeine-on-reproductive-outcomes-in-women.
110. Rumbold, A., P. Middleton, and C. A. Crowther, "Vitamin Supplementation for Preventing Miscarriage," *Cochrane Library*, 2005; (2):Cd004073.
111. Taylor, A. "Extent of the Problem," *BMJ*, 2003; 327(7412):434.
112. Folkehelseinstituttet. "Fødselsstatistikk for 2014," *FHI*, 2015; [updated 11/19/2015]. Available at: https://www.fhi.no/nyheter/2015/fodselsstatistikkfor-2014-publiser/.
113. https://www.cdc.gov/nchs/data/databriefs/db232.pdf.
114. Dunson, D. B., D. D. Baird, and B. Colombo. "Increased Infertility with Age in Men and Women," *Obstetrics & Gynecology*, 2004; 103(1):51–6.
115. Rothman, K. J., L. A. Wise, H. T. Sorensen, A. H. Riis, E. M. Mikkelsen, and E. E. Hatch. "Volitional Determinants and Age-Related Decline in Fecundability: A General Population Prospective Cohort Study in Denmark," *Fertility and Sterility*, 2013; 99(7):1958–64.
116. Bardos, Hercz, Friedenthal, Missmer, and Williams. "A National Survey."
117. Nagoski. *Come as You Are.*

INDEX

Page numbers followed by *f* and *t* refer to figures and tables, respectively.

ABOUT THE TYPE

Typeset in Minion Pro Regular, 11.5/15 pt.

Minion Pro was designed for Adobe Systems by Robert Slimbach in 1990. Inspired by typefaces of the Renaissance, it is both easily readable and extremely functional without compromising its inherent beauty.

Typeset by Scribe Inc., Philadelphia, Pennsylvania.